W9-DIJ-960

CONTENTS

Chapter

Dedication

To my father, Joseph A. Price, without whom this elucidation of the chlorine/atherosclerosis theory with all of its indescribably beneficial implications for greatly increased health and life for many millions of fellow human beings throughout the world would not have been possible. He was indispensably involved with this Chlorine Theory, its experimental proof, its initial dissemination as described in this book and otherwise since its original conception decades ago. Through many, many hours of discussion with me he not only was instrumental in the delineation of basic concepts, but his continual encouragement in spite of adversity and frustrations in presenting such vital, life-saving information to hostile medical/medical research professions and the basically indifferent, if suffering, public over the years has been of incalculable value.

With but little formal education, he possessed the essential prerequisite (lacking in the great majority of members of our basically over-schooled but under-educated society) necessary for participating in true discovery, an open mind. During all the intervening years between the initial presentation of the amazing discovery elucidated herein and his death at the age of 89 in April 13, 1995, and despite never enjoying any of the rewards that were due him, he "kept the faith", knowing that this amazing chlorine/atherosclerosis theory is an idea who "time will (finally) come." After more than 3 decades of continued persistence in purpose of disseminating this amazing information to the needy public, the inexorable wave of history is about to inundate the little minds who have placed multitudes of obstacles in our path to the widespread recognition of the truths contained herein, to the incredible detriment of humanity. As it was best put in a moment of frustration by Mr. George Romney, a very perceptive and insightful former governor or the State of Michigan, "A pox on these petty curs, snapping at the heels of men of accomplishment."

Coronaries/Cholesterol/Chlorine

Eat, Drink And Be Healthy, For Tomorrow You May Dine

Revised Edition

by Joseph M. Price, M.D.

ISBN: 0-515-08825-0

Biographical Sketch

The author of this book, Joseph M. Price, M.D., was born March 21, 1941 in Thetford Township, Genesee County, Michigan. He received his Bachelor of Science degree, "with distinction", from the University of Michigan in 1962. His Doctor of Medicine degree was granted by the University of Michigan Medical School in 1966. After a rotating internship at St. Luke's Hospital in Saginaw, Michigan, Dr. Price was drafted into the U.S. Army Medical Corps, serving a full tour of duty in Vietnam which included a stint as a Battalion Surgeon in the field with the 2/3, 199th Light Infantry Battalion in 1968, seeing "front-line" action during the infamous Tet Offensive. After return to civilian life, Dr. Price practiced full-time Emergency Room medicine for about seven years. Since 1976 he has been in "old-fashioned" solo rural Family Practice in the "Thumb" of Michigan. Dr. Price is Board Certified in the Specialty of Family Practice by the American Board of Family Practice, is active in his local Sanilac County Medical Society and is on the Active Staff of his local hospital. Married in 1974, he is the proud father of 5 children ages 14 to 25. His main hobbies are gardening and growing fruit trees on the family farm where he lives and has his medical office.

Author's Foreword

This is without doubt the most important book you will ever read, because it will likely save your very life. In its original edition (in print for 25 years) it did a good job in presenting my Chlorine Theory of Atherosclerosis in language easily understandable to the medically lay public. Unfortunately, and to the great detriment of millions, this book has been opposed by "Establishment" vested interests at every turn, using every means possible to suppress its lifesaving message.

While in no way obsoleting the original edition and the principles it presents, with the passage of time new evidence and proofs, and, more importantly, new solutions and modes of action have arisen. Therefore it was felt that an "updated" edition would be useful. Accordingly, this revised edition is basically the original text, with only minor changes and additions except for the "Practical Suggestions" chapter which has been almost completely changed to reflect the great advances made over the last couple decades in the availability of very useful home water treatment devices and systems. (It's hard to believe, but in 1969 even the basic, simple activated charcoal filter was not really available for home use!) In order to maintain a sense of authenticity of the original edition as reprinted, any changes of more than minor significance have been put into brackets "[ ]".

What is of most importance in the additional material included is, first of all, detailed advice on what exactly you can (and must) do to protect yourself and your family members from the poisonous chlorine in your drinking water. (May I point out that before the advent of publication of the original edition of this book, chlorine was a medical and public health "sacred cow." Today, as a specific result of this book, almost every water filter manufacturer/retailer emphasizes "Chlorine" first in the list of harmful substances removed by their particular device. In this way I have already made a very significant mark on history.)

As a corollary of showing the reader what actions he needs to take personally to free himself from the fear of atherosclerotic-based heart attack/stroke/ etc., the good news that one does not need to deprive himself of real, good-tasting, natural foods—eggs, beef, pork, lamb, whole milk, etc.—is detailed to some degree.

Next, further proofs of my theory are provided—some based on clinical, epidemiological and demographic evidence, some on classical formal scientific experimentation. (The latter was mainly sponsored by the U.S. Environmental Protection Agency [EPA]. Unfortunately such evidence has been and is being suppressed—but they can't "unwrite" the published papers and the letters in my possession, some reproduced in this new edition.)

Preface

"Give not that which is holy unto the dogs, neither cast ye your pearls before swine, lest they trample them under their feet, and turn again and rend you."
—St. Matthew, 7:6

[The original edition of this book was first published in 1969. Some time thereafter the publishing rights (without pictures) were contracted to a "reprint" publishing firm, and without any advertising or publisher's promotion it became a "secret best seller" with officially over 250,000 copies sold over the years.

When first organizing this revised and updated edition I had intended to basically incorporate newer findings, give support to my claims, and put a description of the opposition to the book and its revolutionary theory as well as plans and projections for the future into the existing text. But it was pointed out to me that one of the great strengths of the original edition was its simple, clear, and easily understandable presentation of fairly complex medical concepts to the medically lay reader.

At this point, I must mention that my detractors have tried to denounce and dismiss the historical basis of my chlorine/atherosclerosis theory as "anecdotal", suggesting that any "legitimate" scientific treatise cannot possibly be valid without citing dozens of references in the medical literature. Furthermore, this "anecdotal" put-down strongly suggests that anything written so that it is understandable by medically lay persons cannot be true. But much of the historical and demographic material referred to in this book is a matter of observation, not readily lending itself to formal "research" and statistical "proofs". If it were otherwise (ie., a matter of orthodox "scientific" research with a review of the antecedent literature pointing to the solution of the problem), the causative chlorine-atherosclerosis relationship would have been evident to third-rate medical researchers three-quarters of a century ago, and the heart attack would have been a mere blip on the record of medical history, instead of being the single major medical problem of the 20th century in "developed" nations. And may I point out that because my chicken experiments represented the absolutely first (and for the greater part of two decades, the only) specific study relating chlorine ingestion to the development of atherosclerosis, there simply was no prior research to which to refer!

While the subject matter of this book is very special, may I point out that it is also unique in another way: Someone once stated, "If you steal from one author it's plagiarism, but if you steal from one hundred it's 'research'". You will note that 99+% of all books written are merely a compendium of what a multitude of other authors have had to say on the subject in question. In contrast, this book is almost 100% new and original. It presents a (now proven) Theory that was first presented to the world in the original (1969 copyright) edition of this book. It copies nobody's ideas, claims or concepts. This book may be opinionated, rude, imperious, even downright nasty at times. But you will find it lays it on the line, tells nothing but the unvarnished truth no matter whose ox gets gored, pulls no punches to avoid upsetting the "powers that be", and is, I sincerely hope, always interesting and above all, informative.

If by the time you finish this book you have not decided to make major changes in your life-style regarding what kind of water you drink (and rewarding yourself with the good foods you have in well-intentioned ignorance of the true facts been avoiding), I will have failed my purpose in writing such. But I have a feeling that you will be entering a new time of understanding, freedom from the irrational fear of cholesterol and heart attacks, health, and renewed enjoyment of life including truly satisfying nutrition!

It is sad that so many well-intentioned folks in an ill-advised attempt to preserve their health have adopted artificial, chemical-laden, "low-cholesterol" foods (margarine, ersatz bacon, fake eggs, and so forth) as mainstays of their diets. They have foolishly made sacrifices, in a sense a Spartan "eating to live" instead of "living to eat", unnecessarily avoiding really pleasurable, healthy,

9

natural foods (such as red meats, eggs, butter, whole milk, etc.). Such dietary asceticism would be admirable if it were based on truthful principles. Unfortunately, such dietary changes are useless (in preventing atherosclerosis, heart attacks and strokes) and may actually be detrimental (more cancer from the unnatural chemicals). Yes, you can "have your cake and eat it". As long as you 100% of the time drink only chlorine-free water, you can eat anything without fear of heart attack and related diseases.

Eggs (any way you want 'em), sausage, real bacon, toast with real butter, real butter melted over vegetables, beef roast, pork roast, ham, pork chops, leg o' lamb, lamb chops, whole milk, real cream, and on and on and on. These are not only good, natural foods, real foods, but they are good for you! Avoid the chlorine in water and enjoy!]

LINUS PAULING INSTITUTE of SCIENCE and MEDICINE

440 Page Mill Road, Palo Alto, California 94306
Telephone: (415) 327-4064

4 January 1984

Dr. Joseph M. Price
4640 East Sanilac Road
Carsonville, MI 48419

Dear Dr. Price:

I apologize for the delay in answering your letter, the result of my having been traveling.

I have read your book with interest, and also your letter. I am sorry to learn about how much trouble you have been having with the authorities.

If there is any way in which I might help you, please let me know.

I have thought about the question of possible mechanisms of action of the chlorine and chlorinated water. Probably the chlorine ingested in drinking chlorinated water would be reduced to chloride in the gut, and would not get into the bloodstream. It is thus likely that the principal effect would be on the ingested food. Presumably this effect would be the oxidation of reducing agents in the food.

One possibility is that vitamin C would be destroyed. The median intake of vitamin C in the food of Americans was shown by a survey a number of years ago to be 49 mg per day. The amount of chlorine in the drinking water is unlikely to destroy this much vitamin C. Moreover, chickens manufacture much larger amounts of vitamin C in their own cells, and, although the amount of chlorine added to the water in your experiment was rather high, it is unlikely that it would have destroyed much of the vitamin C, and your chickens do not seem to have shown signs of scurvy.

On the other hand, the median intake of vitamin E is much smaller, probably 15 I.U. (15 mg of d,l-alpha-tocopherol), and a good bit of the vitamin E in the food might be destroyed by chlorine in the drinking water, especially since the stoichiometric factor is rather large. Possibly this destruction of vitamin E by chlorinated water would be a factor.

Sincerely,

Linus Pauling

LP:dm

11

UNITED STATES ENVIRONMENTAL PROTECTION AGENCY
WASHINGTON, D.C. 20460

MAR 2 4 1986

OFFICE OF
RESEARCH AND DEVELOPMENT

Honorable Donald W. Riegle, Jr.
United States Senate
Washington, D.C. 20510

Dear Senator Riegle:

I am writing to you in response to your letter dated February 25, 1986, in which you forwarded Dr. Joseph Price's letter discussing the relationship between chlorine and cardiovascular disease. The U.S. Environmental Protection Agency (EPA) is concerned about the possible health effects of chlorine and other drinking water disinfectants and published regulations to control disinfectant by-products in 1979. These regulations are in the process of being revised and expanded to include, if appropriate, disinfectant residues. They are scheduled to be proposed in 1988. The scope of these regulations will be to protect the public from all the possible health effects of the use of disinfectants including cardiovascular disease.

In addition to the regulatory activities, the EPA's Office of Health Research is conducting specific animal and human studies on the relationship between chlorine and cardiovascular disease. Specifically, we are conducting studies with chlorine, chlorine dioxide and chloramine in both rabbits and pigeons to determine the dose-response effects of these chemicals on the formation of atherosclerotic plaques and cardiovascular disease. Concurrently, we are conducting human clinical studies under controlled conditions to determine the effect of these compounds on serum cholesterol levels, blood pressure and other clinical parameters related to heart disease. Finally, we are conducting an epidemiological study in Wisconsin to determine the effects of chlorine in drinking water on cardiovascular disease in a human population.

We believe this is a strong research program, designed to assess potential risks associated with the use of disinfectants in drinking water. This research directly supports EPA's mission.

In response to Dr. Price's charge that EPA is "stonewalling," I would like to point out that EPA funded the studies by Dr. Revis cited in Dr. Price's letter and that these studies were published with EPA's approval. I believe EPA's regulatory and research activities demonstrate that EPA takes this issue seriously.

Thank you for your interest in this topic.

Sincerely,

Donald O. Ehreth
Acting Assistant Administrator
for Research and Development

12

UNITED STATES ENVIRONMENTAL PROTECTION AGENCY
OFFICE OF RESEARCH AND DEVELOPMENT
HEALTH EFFECTS RESEARCH LABORATORY
CINCINNATI, OHIO 45268

January 15, 1987

Joseph M. Price, M.D.
Carsonville, MI 48419

Dear Dr. Price:

Pursuant to the topic of our telephone conversation of December 15, 1986, I am writing to you requesting sample copies of your writings regarding the involvement of chlorinated drinking water in the etiology of atherosclerosis.

As I outlined to you in our telephone conversation, my research with non-human primates and other laboratory animal species resulted in observations and data which indicates that ingestion of chlorine (hypochlorite) treated water causes depression of serum "High Density Lipoprotein" (HDL) bound cholesterol, shifting cholesterol binding to the "Low density" form (LDL). The involvement of HDL in protection against Coronary Heart Disease (CHD) and the role of LDL in development of arterial atherosclerotic lesions, I am sure you agree, is an established medical fact.

We are now beginning to disassemble and understand this phenomenon on the molecular and cellular level, and I believe, we will have shortly validated proof for the mechanisms involved.

I understand, your initial and seminal work with chickens in connecting atherosclerotic lesions with Cl_2-disinfected water had little acceptance by peer review. No wonder, at the time of your research, none of the modern concepts of lipoprotein metabolism, nor the methods invoked in our studies existed. So much more reason exists, I believe, to appreciate the acuity of your observations, and intuitive accuracy in identifying the causative agent of this "whodunit" pathological phenomenon.

I am intrigued therefore, to read your writings and more importantly, to see any of your experimental records, if available. In particular I am interested by any observations you may have made regarding the dose responsiveness and timing of onset of plaque formation in chickens. I assure that any printed matter or experimental data record you may send me will be promptly returned to you. I will be much obliged for your reply.

Sincerely yours,

J. Peter Bercz, Ph.D., DABCC
Toxicologist
Target Organ Toxicology Branch
Toxicology and Microbiology Division

13

Chapter 1

A Full Scale Epidemic

The United States is in the midst of an unprecedented disease epidemic. The word "epidemic" brings to mind horrifying images of infectious diseases sweeping a nation. This situation obviously does not exist in the U.S. today. Nevertheless, each year heart attacks and strokes kill and maim many times the number of persons afflicted by all the serious infectious diseases combined.

Just about everyone knows somebody, relative or friend, who has had or died from a heart attack or stroke. These two disease entities, along with cancer, are so widespread and of such importance in America today that the Congress of the United States has appropriated many millions of dollars to set up nationwide regional health centers devoted exclusively to medical research on and treatment of these afflictions. This constitutes the largest and most ambitious medical project, in terms, of manpower, facilities, and expense, ever attempted in recorded history.

[Cardiovascular and cerebrovascular diseases ("coronary heart disease and stroke") together constitute the main as yet uncontrolled disease processes afflicting mankind today. [In 1988 William P. Castelli, M.D., Director of the famous Framingham (Mass.) Heart Study stated "Coronary disease and atherosclerosis account for half of the reasons that people die today']

*William P. Castelli, M.D., "Cholesterol as a Cardiac Risk Factor", Doctors Mart, Vol. 12,#4, 1988.

The coronary heart attack (the same disease process is known under several other names, such as "coronary thrombosis", or "myocardial infarction", but in this presentation we will generally use the term "heart attack") is by a substantial margin the number-one killer in the United States today. More than one-half million Americans die each year of heart attacks. But the true size of the problem is not properly conveyed with such black-and-white statistics. In addition to deaths, one must not forget the vast toll of nonfatal heart attacks—the costs of medical care, loss of wages, the incalculable physical and mental anguish of the patients and his family, etc. Even if the victim does not die, the effects on himself and his loved ones may be absolutely devastating nonetheless. From a broader point of view the loss of productivity of survivors is tremendous—as loss for our nation as a whole. It is in all truthfulness a full scale epidemic.

Chapter 2

The Heart Attack

Especially if you are a middle-aged man, you are probably a bit more than a little concerned about this problem. What really is a heart attack? You may be wondering in the back of your mind what's its like to have a heart attack. More to the point, what the chances that I am going to have a heart attack and hopefully, is there anything I can do to help protect myself against suffering one?

Let us consider these questions one at a time.

Everyone knows that a person who has had a heart attack has had something bad suddenly happen to his heart and as a result he may die. But for the reader to really understand what is going to be explained later regarding the final solution to this killer, a little preliminary explanation is in order regarding what really happens *in the heart*.

First of all, it is necessary to become acquainted at least superficially with a few facts about the anatomy of the heart. The heart is an amazing hollow muscle about the size of your clenched fist which serves the life-sustaining function of pumping blood to all parts of the body. It starts beating a few weeks after conception while the child is still in its mother's womb and continues unabated until death. The heart, like any other muscle in the body, must constantly receive a flow of blood carrying food and oxygen in order to live. What is not understood by the vast majority of non-medical persons is that in the human being the heart muscle itself cannot use any of the blood contained within its pumping chambers. Instead the supply of blood to the heart muscle comes entirely from two little vessels, called coronary (heart) arteries, which arise from the main artery of the body, the aorta, run along the outside surface of the heart and then enter into the heart muscle to feed it.

Since these two little arteries are the *only* source of blood to the heart muscle, when one of them (or one of their branches) suddenly becomes blocked off, the portion of the heart muscle supplied by the involved artery dies. This death of a portion of the heart muscle is called in medical terminology a "myocardial infarction" or in common language a "heart attack". If the part of the heart muscle which dies is small, the dead portion will be gradually replaced by scar tissue and the patient is likely to recover. If a large part of the heart muscle is affected, death may come within minutes or hours, usually the result of an "arrhythmia" or irregular heart beat; or it may be the result of other complications manifested most commonly during the first two weeks of convalescence.

Now that we understand, at least in general terms, what happens in the heart itself during a heart attack let us consider what happens to the victim. What does he feel and what is it like to have a heart attack? The person who is having a heart attack usually experiences the sudden onset of a severe crushing, compressing type of mid-chest pain which may shoot down the arm and sometimes up the neck, especially on the left side. This pain is often accompanied by a feeling of imminent disaster with associated cold sweat, nausea, weakness and sometimes shortness of breath. Many victims of heart attacks give a history of intermittent chest pains beginning a few days or more before the acute infarct (premonitory pain.) A physical examination and electrocardiogram done by a physician at this time usually will *not* reveal significant abnormalities. After the actual heart attack has taken place (chest pain, etc., as above) electrocardiograms and certain blood tests (enzyme studies) ordered by the physician can be used to confirm the diagnosis and in some instances will give an indication of the probable prognosis, ie., chance of survival.

Now that we have an idea about what it is like to have a heart attack and understand that it is due to sudden blocking off of one of the little arteries carrying blood to the heart muscle, the next question that arises is what causes the sudden occlusion ("blocking off")? While the actual total occlusion of a coronary artery which results in an acute heart attack takes place suddenly, it only occurs in previously diseased arteries affected by a pathological process known as *atherosclerosis*. Atherosclerosis is a particular kind of "hardening of the arteries" characterized by the gradual accumulation of certain fatty substances embedded in the inner wall of the arteries, slowly making the lumen ("opening") smaller and smaller. This process can be compared, for the sake of clarity, to the gradual deposition of lime scales on the inner surfaces of hot water pipes, except that in the arteries, the process is further complicated by the body's reaction to the deposit of foreign material. The deposits of fatty material which result from this process are called *atheromas* and appear grossly as raised yellow-colored plaques. A heart attack occurs when spontaneous bleeding in or around an atheromatous plaque causes a blood clot to form which then blocks the blood flow through a coronary artery, hence the term "coronary thrombosis". There could not be a heart attack if the coronary arteries were not partially closed by atheromatous plaques.

You are probably wondering if there is any way to tell if your own coronary arteries are in good condition or if they are partially occluded with atherosclerotic plaques and liable to sudden occlusion with resulting heart attack. The answer is that there is no safe, noninvasive way to prove that the coronary arteries are definitely in good condition. A person may look and feel fine, his physician may pronounce him physically sound after performing a thorough examination, including an electrocardiogram, and even after stress testing, only to suddenly collapse with an acute heart attack going out the door! On the other hand, angina pectoris, a syndrome of intermittent chest pains usually precipitated by exercise, emotional stress, or other factors such as exposure to cold, is *prima facie* evidence of coronary insufficiency, ie., the coronary arteries so narrowed by atherosclerosis that the heart does not receive enough blood to support its functions during certain periods of greater need. So while a man may have advanced coronary atherosclerosis and be "ripe" for a heart attack without any symptoms whatsoever, the presence of angina pectoris usually means that there are quite advanced changes present in the arteries and a heart attack is a definite, ever present threat.

With reference to the asymptomatic group, there are a series of factors which are correlated with a predisposition to heart attacks. These include:

1. Male sex
2. Cigarette smoking
3. Elevated blood pressure
4. Middle age or older
5. High blood levels of cholesterol or "LDL's (low density lipoproteins)
6. Diabetes mellitus
7. Obesity
8. Low levels of physical activity
9. Family history of heart attacks
10. Shortness of stature
11. "Soft" drinking water
12. Others

If you live in a "developed" nation, especially America or Europe, the more items on this list which apply to you the more likely you are to be a prime candidate for a heart attack.

You will notice that number one on the list is "male sex". The typical heart attack victim is an overweight, middle-aged man who is physically inactive and smokes cigarettes. But this stereotype leaves us with several important questions unanswered. For example, do women get heart attacks? From the medical propaganda in the news media, one would think that the answer is, "Yes, of course." And I have had young women (in their 20s) come into my office asking for me to take their "cholesterol levels," telling me that they don't eat eggs or read meat anymore all because they are afraid of clogging up their arteries and having a heart attack! The answer to this question is a very qualified "yes," that women do indeed get heart attacks but only after the menopause, unless they have some other serious complicating disease such as diabetes and/or hypertension or some other disease entity, such as the fairly rare systemic lupus erythematosis. So except in the case of these unusual circumstances, pre-menopausal women (usually between about the ages of 12 and 50) are essentially immune to the development of atherosclerosis/clogging up of the arteries and subsequent heart attacks and strokes based on such disease process. This "immunity" is thought to be related in some way to secretion of estrogens (female sex hormones) and ceases to exist when the ovaries (female sex glands) are removed or stop active functioning. In fact, administration of synthetic estrogens to men with strong predispositions to heart attacks has been suggested, but has failed to gain wide acceptance for obvious reasons.

Do young men or even children ever get heart attacks? Surprisingly enough, it is a misconception to think of the heart attack as a disease only of middle-aged and old men. While it is true that the disease is seen mainly in these groups, heart attacks have become more common in younger age groups in recent years. We are now seeing heart attacks in apparently healthy men in their 30s and, under special circumstances of genetic abnormalities, even fatal heart attacks in children. As will be described in some detail later, the underlying disease process of atherosclerosis may start in early childhood.

By now it should be clear that a heart attack is but the end result of a more general disease process in which deposits are built up in the inside lining of arteries. It only seems logical that this buildup does not occur suddenly, e.g. overnight. Does it take months? Years? The facts are that while an actual heart attack is one of the most dramatic events in medicine, the underlying disease process of the development of atherosclerosis is quite the opposite. The infiltration of the artery walls begins in most cases at least 10 to 20 years before any overt symptoms present themselves. But it is important to realize that not all men in any one age group have arteries in the same condition of blockage. Some men die at the age of 45 of heart attacks while other men of identical age may have youthful, clean arteries good for another 45 years. Even today in "developed" countries, some men die in advanced old age with but absolutely minimal evidence of arterial disease.

Chapter 3

Strokes

Thus far we have centered our attention on the coronary heart attack. As I hope is quite clear by now, when atherosclerosis involves the coronary (heart) arteries, it gives rise to heart attacks. But atherosclerosis, that form of "hardening of the arteries" which results from the building-up of fatty deposits on the inside lining of arteries, may occur almost anywhere in the body's arterial system. As a general rule, it may be said that the signs and symptoms resulting from an advanced atherosclerotic process involving an artery are the signs and symptoms of lack of blood supply to the particular organ(s) supplied.

When the arteries feeding the brain are affected by atherosclerosis, the stage is set for the occurrence of that other great killer and maimer of modern civilization, the stroke. A stroke occurs when the blood supply to a part of the brain is compromised. With loss of a source of free-flowing blood to nourish it, the affected part of the brain may die. Unfortunately, in contrast to the heart which is fairly unspecialized and can "make up" for heart tissue destroyed by a heart attack with surviving tissue, brain tissue tends to be highly specialized and therefore when certain parts of the brain die functions related to such areas are oftentimes lost forever—hence, the paralyses, loss of ability to talk, read, or to understand speech or the written word, etc. following strokes. The two great subdivisions of stroke are the cerebral hemorrhage (bleeding from a vessel into the brain substance) and the cerebral thrombosis (a blood clot blocking a cerebral/brain vessel which has been narrowed by atherosclerotic plaque. With a few exceptions (e.g. congenital berry aneurysm) the great majority of strokes have the process of atherosclerosis as the underlying cause—either by weakening artery walls with consequent rupture and bleeding into the brain or by narrowing the lumen of arteries in the brain predisposing to sudden occlusion by a blood clot. The so-called "small stroke" most commonly results from the breaking off of small portions of atheromas and their blocking off of small cerebral (brain) vessels.

Chapter 4

Other Atherosclerotic Disease Entities

Although heart attack and stroke are the two immensely important end results of atherosclerosis, there are several other clinical entities secondary to the same disease process. For instance, if the arteries supplying the brain are progressively narrowed due to growing atheromas, but without an acute episode of occlusion or bleeding which would cause a stroke, there is evidenced signs of chronic cerebrovascular insufficiency—spells of dizziness, transient paralyses, forgetfulness, and loss of mental acuity. A fairly common form of "senility" is the result of multiple small or "mini"-strokes secondary to the breaking off of small pieces of atherosclerotic plaque which then clog arteries feeding the brain. If instead the atherosclerosis affects mainly the arteries to the legs ("peripheral vascular insufficiency") we see evident the syndromes related to peripheral artery disease—intermittent claudication (pain in the calf muscles on walking but relieved by rest) or even gangrene of the toes, feet or even legs (seen most commonly in diabetics). Aneurysms of the abdominal aorta (great dilatations of part of the body's main artery which may burst resulting in sudden death from internal hemorrhage) are almost all secondary to weakening of the vessel walls from atheroma formation. Finally, we should not forget that a very significant number of cases of physiologic sexual impotency in the male is due to atherosclerosis blocking off the normal blood supply to the sexual organs. A psychologically normal man who is free from atherosclerosis and serious neurological disorders such as diabetic neuropathy should be sexually potent well into his 70s or 80s! There are a few other less common disorders and manifestations related to atherosclerosis which are not of sufficient prevalence or importance to discuss at this time.

From these brief descriptions it can be realized that atherosclerosis is the basic pathological process behind many of the most devastating diseases of this century.

22

In particular, it is the underlying cause of the majority of the chronic diseases which are ravaging the land and against which present-day medical science can do but little.

To summarize, the disease process of atherosclerosis is the basis for:

1. *Heart attacks* (myocardial infarction, coronary thrombosis, etc..) and angina pectoris (heart pains).

2. *Strokes*

3. Peripheral artery disease (including the symptoms of intermittent claudication)

4. Aneurysms of the aorta (and other arteries)

5. Senility/dementia of old age due to "mini"-strokes

6. Male sexual impotency due to vascular insufficiency

7. Miscellaneous other syndromes

Chapter 5

The Cholesterol Theory

The next consideration which quite naturally arises is what exactly is this special form of "hardening of the arteries" called atherosclerosis? Is it known why the arteries get clogged up with fatty deposits? Let me here and now make the flat statement that modern medical science does *not* acknowledge a definite known causal factor for atherosclerosis. (Despite the impression left by articles in the lay press, and even in many medical journal articles!) In fact, there are strong disagreements among medical scientists as to such basic knowledge as the exact mechanism of accumulation of lipids in the inner linings of arteries, much less is there any agreement about the underlying cause of such deposition. The only things that are known as to the cause of atherosclerosis are certain *correlations*, and a correlation does *not* in any way imply causation. (A correlation, in simple terms, means that two different things tend to exist together but does not necessarily mean that one causes the other. As an absurd example, I am told that there can be demonstrated a close correlation between the amount of bananas imported into England and the birth rate there. Less facetiously, and of some importance because it demonstrates a significant point regarding correlations between atherosclerosis and various factors—as will be explained in more detail later—is the fantastic correlation between the number of telephones per unit of population and the cardiac (heart) death rate. This correlation is more striking than the correlation between atherosclerosis, heart attacks and any of the alleged dietary factors.)

While it has been acknowledged that a correlation exists between the development of atherosclerosis and such varied factors as age, sex, genetic constitution, endocrine balance, psychic state, drugs, exercise, occupation and climate, most interest and research in the field of the study of atherogenesis (the cause of atherosclerosis) has centered around a fatty chemical substance called *cholesterol*.

Despite the widespread feeling that cholesterol is some sore of evil ogre, a substance that God by mistake put into good-tasting foods to kill human beings, the fact of the matter is that cholesterol is a lipid (fatty) substance which occurs in all animal cells and is absolutely essential to life of all animals. It is needed by the body as the chemical starting point for many essential compounds. For example, the vital steroidal hormones, which include the basic male and female sex hormones, can be made only from cholesterol. The human brain itself is made up of a very high percentage of cholesterol.

The body's cholesterol comes from two sources. First of all, cholesterol is so important that regardless of dietary intake the body will make up necessary cholesterol itself from simpler compounds. In fact, the body's homeostasis with regards to cholesterol is so important that it regulates cholesterol in cells closer than about any other compound. (In view of this it seems amazing that our medical scientists in their ignorance have managed to convince the vast majority of medically lay persons of the inherent dangers and evilness of cholesterol, whether the level in the bloodstream or in good foods.) Secondly, a certain amount of cholesterol is taken into the body whenever certain foods of animal origin (e.g. fatty meats, milk, eggs, butter, etc.) are eaten. This dietary cholesterol is *not* some sort of insidious, slow poison! As the body maintains its cholesterol homeostasis, if it is able to get cholesterol from dietary sources, it simply does not have to make its own otherwise.

There are several reasons why modern medical researchers have centered most of their heart research investigations around the substance cholesterol, and have assigned it such importance—many medical scientists point an accusing finger at cholesterol as *the* primary causative agent in atherogenesis. First, it has been known for many decades that atheromatous plaques wherever they form are composed chemically mainly of cholesterol. In fact, some claim that an atheroma is essentially an inflammatory response of the body to a cholesterol deposit. Secondly, lesions very similar to human atheromas may be produced at will in certain species of animals by feeding them diets high in cholesterol. Finally, it is thought that there is a correlation between blood cholesterol levels in men and their likelihood of developing one of the atheromatous diseases, e.g. heart attack or stroke. In certain families there is a rare genetic (inherited) defect which results in affected members having fantastically high blood cholesterol levels. Children in these families have been known to die from heart attacks before they reach eight years of age.

It would seem that if cholesterol is the primary cause of atherosclerosis one could avoid heart attacks and strokes by avoiding foods high in cholesterol. Is this as valid statement? It is true that this point of view has many influential proponents. The most widely accepted theory holds that it is the excessive consumption of foods containing cholesterol that predisposes to atherosclerosis and its sequelae. As a result of the widespread acceptance of this cholesterol theory there has been an informal [Also formal as of 1987 with the creation of the "National Cholesterol Education Program" of the "National Heart, Lung, and Blood Institute".] nation-wide campaign on for the last few years to discourage the "excessive" consumption of foods high in fats and cholesterol. As a corollary of this, researchers have discovered that certain types of fat, called "polyunsaturated" and found primarily in vegetable oils, have a vague antagonistic effect in the body on the "saturated" animal fats which are high in cholesterol. Witness the commercialization of this finding in ads and on TV—"So-and-so margarine, highest in polyunsaturated fats!" [But in 1994 the chief of nutrition at Harvard University medical school has gone into print pointing out that margarines contain artificial—not found in nature—"trans"-fats produced by the hydrogenation process that are worse than saturated, resulting in 20,000 extra heart attacks per year in the U.S.!]

Many "experts" in the field believe that if by diet, drugs or by other means one can lower his blood cholesterol levels he has significantly reduced his chances of developing a heart attack or stroke. And a series of (very expensive) new drugs that lower the level of blood lipids (fatty substances) including cholesterol in the hope of delaying or eliminating heart attacks and strokes have become available in recent years.

Chapter 6

Is The Cholesterol Theory Valid?

"Well-organized ignorance often passes, unfortunately, for wisdom"

—Anonymous

In spite of the remarks made in the previous chapter, this belief in the possible avoidance of atherosclerosis by dietary manipulation is by no means universal. It has been emphasized by a minority of researchers that *no* direct evidence exists to prove that lowering of blood cholesterol by any method possible will actually decrease the risk of coronary heart disease or stroke, or even affect the underlying atherosclerosis. In fact, the U.S. Food and Drug Administration has taken this stand in its regulation of advertising to physicians of the new serum lipid (cholesterol and triglyceride) lowering drugs. [This last sentence was written 25 years ago. Today with several newer lipid-lowering drugs, the pharmaceutical companies *still* have not been able to show that their drugs favorably affect mortality (death) rate from heart attacks and have to state so in their package inserts for prescribing physicians!]

Although as causal relationship between cholesterol and heart attacks and strokes (the cholesterol theory of atherosclerosis) has not been proven, the circumstantial evidence may seem pretty convincing. Is there any evidence for the other view, ie., the cholesterol theory may not be the complete story? Indeed there is. In discussing this other side of the picture it should be remembered that modern medical science hates to admit that it does not know the answer to a problem. So it proposes a hypothetical solution—really an educated guess. Fair enough—one needs a starting point from which to proceed. Unfortunately, for lack of anything better the cholesterol hypothesis has attained almost the status

27

of an established and definitely proven theory—not because anything has been proven but rather because it fills what would otherwise be an intolerable scientific vacuum.

The cholesterol theory has become so thoroughly accepted as God-given truth that many otherwise intelligent, scientifically-oriented, insightful medical authorities explain away in a most illogical manner any evidence which would cast a shadow of a doubt on its "unquestionable" validity. The reason for this appallingly unscientific attitude is that rejection of the cholesterol theory would require the substitution of a presumably more acceptable hypothesis. Needless to say, the cholesterol theory, imperfect [actually utterly erroneous] as it may be, is acknowledged by the orthodox medical profession to be the only possible plausible one presented so far [prior to publication of the original edition of this book in 1969]. If the cholesterol theory would be discarded and not replaced by something more reasonable, medicine would be admitting total impotency against modern mankind's major killers. This, as implied strongly before, is completely unacceptable.

[I wrote the above in composing the original edition of this book when I was only 28 years old, just returned from service in Vietnam as a combat infantry battalion surgeon. Since that time 25 years, a full quarter of a century, has passed and at least 12 million Americans have died needlessly from heart attacks alone in this period of time. In that span of time I have "kept the faith", have tried to make this wonderful, lifesaving knowledge known to all I could by whatever means available to me, oftentimes at a personal cost to me financially, professionally, and otherwise that would make a normal man shudder. Over a quarter of a million copies of the original edition of this book have been published, millions have heard of my name and my Chlorine Theory from the book, quotes in advertising brochures, lectures I have given, and television appearances I have made over the years. At this point in time there is not a single manufacturer or seller of home water filter/purification units who does not emphasize that his product removes chlorine, such chlorine being a sacred cow before the publication of the first edition of this book and regarded as important to be removed from drinking water only because of the facts presented in this book! At present

one out of every seven residents of California drinks bottled or filtered water, with essentially every one of them at least subliminally aware of the dangers of chlorine. Is it any wonder that rates of heart attacks have been gradually falling since the original publication of this book?

Yet I and my theory remain essentially unknown to the orthodox medical profession, and I languish professionally making my living in a dirt-poor, obscure rural area as a solo family practitioner, the least prestigious and lowest paid medical specialty. Needless to say, try as I may I have a very hard time thinking charitable thoughts when I hear of a rich city invasive cardiology specialist dropping dead of a heart attack—"physician, heal thyself". I'm only human and many times over the years I have had to ask why has my Chlorine Theory, the single most important medical discovery of the 20th century, been ignored by the medical profession and I denied my just rewards (oh, hell, any rewards)?

I have been well aware since the very beginning of the chemical companies "conspiracy of silence" against my book and its Chlorine Theory. After all, when I was first trying to get the book published (by *anyone*) in the 1960s the lawyer who was going to do wonders with it pulled out suddenly admitting chemical company pressure.

More recently I have realized that the medical/medical research professions refusal to even entertain much less espouse my cause is based on certain very strong fundamentals. It should be obvious that medical doctors/researchers who have made their careers covering decades based on the presumptive validity of the cholesterol theory are not going to possess open minds regarding a theory apt to destroy these careers, their work of these past couple decades, their very livelihood! Billions of taxpayers dollars have gone into useless (and actually very harmful because of its effect in suppressing my Chlorine Theory) heart disease research over many years. And the beneficiaries of this largess are suddenly going to say that they were wrong all along, that those billions of dollars were totally wasted by them in useless, meaningless "research" and that millions of Americans have died of heart attacks needlessly in the meantime?

But more disconcerting even than the above is my more recent realization that not only among the medical/medical research professions but also with regards to the general public the cholesterol theory (as mentioned above, a *simplistic* theory only conceived of in the first place and then presented to the public because medical leaders and spokesmen were unwilling to admit the truth that they really didn't know the cause of atherosclerosis) has attained the status of a true *mass delusion*. To explain a bit: in 1841 Charles Mackay wrote a book entitled "Extraordinary Popular Delusions and the Madness of Crowds" detailing certain great mass delusions to that point in time, e.g. Tulipmania, the Mississippi Scheme, The South Sea Bubble, the Crusades and witch hunts. As he said, "Every Age has its peculiar folly, some scheme, project or fantasy into which it plunges—". More recently James P. Hogan put it concisely, "Periodically societies are seized by collective delusions that take on lives of their own, where all facts are swept aside that fail to conform to the expectations of what has become a self-sustaining reality". (Omni, June 1993, p.34)

I propose that the cholesterol theory of atherosclerosis is one of our present day fantasies, a classical *mass delusion* entered into by the top minds of our medical and medical research professions, which has now filtered down through and has encompassed the entire professions and to a great degree even the general public! It has become a self-sustaining mass delusion, feeding on itself *ad infinitum* with no end or reckoning in sight. Economic mass delusions eventually collapse when the money runs out. How can I (an individual medical doctor and a "clinician" at that, among more than 300,000 physicians in the United States alone) with my Chlorine Theory prevail against a mass delusion "where(in) all facts are swept aside that fail to conform to the expectations of what has become a self-sustaining reality"? After 25 years of trying I cannot answer that. I'll just keep plugging along like I am doing right now re-writing this book.]

The considerable evidence against the acceptance of the cholesterol theory as the final word on the subject will now be discussed in some detail. The following considerations, I'm sure you'll agree, are quite convincing in themselves.

If all human beings in the world were, and always had been, uniformly subject to heart attacks and strokes at the same prevalence as found in the United States today, the hope of finding a definitive solution to the problem of atherosclerosis would be dim indeed. For if the above were true we would probably have to accept atherosclerosis as an inevitable part of the aging process. Fortunately, this is not the case at all. Even staunch proponents of the classical cholesterol theory realize that atherosclerosis is a *disease* process which is by no means universal and at least theoretically capable of being retarded and possibly even reversed.

Today in the United States men outnumber women in total heart disease by more than one-third; until approximately 1930 the rates were about the same. The only logical explanation is that since about 1930 coronary heart disease has been affecting men, who before then had been almost as immune as premenopausal women are. That is to say that the heart attack, while occurring before 1930, only reached sufficient proportions to affect statistical tables about then. This would tend to imply that some environmental consideration of supreme importance in the etiology (causation) of atherosclerosis began to affect men in the early part of this century. (Remember that 10 to 20 years of increasing atherosclerosis precedes clinical manifestations.) This could not be cholesterol because cholesterol has been with man as long as there has been man.

I have just introduced the critically important concept that coronary heart disease and other manifestations of atherosclerosis were essentially unknown before the present century, and therefore these disease processes must have an underlying causal agent of rather modern origin. Are there other historical facts which support this contention? Angina pectoris, the intermittent chest pains which usually imply narrowing of the coronary (heart) arteries by atherosclerosis and oftentimes precedes full-blown heart attacks, was first described only as recently as 1768. And not only was it an exceedingly rare disease for the century and a half following this description but the cases described during this period were not necessarily due to an underlying atherosclerotic process—even today it is an undisputable fact that angina pectoris may rarely be the result of some other disease process such as syphilitic involvement of the base of the aorta or anemia of an origin. The non-atheromatous instances of angina pectoris are exceedingly rare, but then so was the syndrome of angina pectoris itself until some years into this century.

Now let us consider the heart attack itself. The coronary heart attack, which is almost exclusively the end result of atherosclerosis of the coronary (heart) arteries, was completely unknown until early in this century. Hard to believe? Yes, it sure is. I'll be the first to admit that most present-day physicians will immediately challenge this statement. But the pure and simple facts are that the first clinical description of coronary thrombosis (another term essentially synonymous with "heart attack") was made as recently as 1912. The great Canadian-American physician Sir William Osler did not mention the existence of the entity in lectures on heart diseases in 1910. And most amazingly, the world-famous heart specialist Dr. Paul Dudley White, who treated President Eisenhower for his heart attack in the early 1950's, did not see his *first* case of myocardial infarction (once again, another term essentially synonymous with "heart attack") until after 1920!! [In 1966 L. Michaels was honest enough to state with reference to coronary thrombosis before 1912: "The possibility must be considered that it (the heart attack) had been almost non-existent rather than prevalent but unrecognized". Michaels, L., "Aetiology of Coronary Heart Disease: An Historical Approach." British Heart Journal, vol. 28, p258-264, 1966.]

Now that I have presented you with historical facts (which may be verified in any good medical library) debunking the concept that atherosclerosis and its clinical manifestations such as the heart attack and stroke are as old as mankind, what is there to say about the role of cholesterol?

Let me make the statement that while cholesterol may be one of many contributing factors to the development of atherosclerosis and its complications, it certainly is not sufficient alone—it is not the factor. The evidence for this point of view is substantial. We should first consider a finding closely related to the facts just described: through careful investigation of the literature it has been shown that in England at the end of the 19th century almost one-third of the population consumed dietary fats in amounts which must be considered excessive by present-day standards, and yet heart attacks and other evidences of atherosclerosis were non-existent! Another most impressive finding is that atherosclerotic heart disease has always been unknown in China—700,000,000 people and no heart attacks! And don't let anyone explain this away by saying that it proves that cholesterol is therefore all-important because the Chinese consume very little dietary fat. While the peasants have always lived on basically vegetarian diets, many of the traditional dishes of the higher social classes who have been able to afford it are nauseatingly fatty. Yet atherosclerosis has been as non-existent among the well-to-do as with the Chinese peasants.

While atherosclerosis and its consequences are practically absent among most primitive peoples of the world, there is no better example of high dietary fat intake coupled with the absence of atherosclerosis than seen among the Eskimos. The dietary fat intake of traditional Eskimos is simply hard to believe—a single adult may eat several pounds of blubber at a sitting. This fantastic dietary pattern is followed for a lifetime—and yet no heart attacks or strokes from atherosclerosis. [More recently (1988) there had been a flap about Eskimos being protected from atherosclerosis by their intake of "omega-3-polyunsaturated fatty acids" from eating cold-water fish. (e.g. Bang HO, Dyerberg J, "Lipid Metabolism and Ischemic Heart Disease in Greenland Eskimos", Adv. Nutr. Res., 3: 1-22, 1980. Kromhout, D, et al, "The Inverse Relation Between Fish Consumption and 20-Year Mortality From Coronary Heart Disease", New England J. Med., 312: 1205-1209, May 9, 1985.) Almost immediately following these (unsubstantiated) claims published in the New England Journal of Medicine the drug hucksters were out peddling their wares. As could almost be expected, more recent studies now suggest that men (non-Eskimos, of course, and presumably ingesting chlorinated water) ingesting these dietary fats may end up with increased levels of the portion of blood cholesterol (LDLs) thought most correlated with development of atherosclerosis!] If there were no other evidence than Eskimos (those following old-fashioned lifestyle patterns) being entirely free of atherosclerosis and heart attacks, any thinking man would still question the cholesterol (dietary fat) theory. Nevertheless, there is still considerably more evidence to raise doubts in our minds.

For instance, if you want something a little nearer to home, we have that, too. A few years ago there was an article in a popular magazine about a small town called Roseto in the hills of Pennsylvania. The people in this town, of Italian descent, tended to be obese and eat a diet abnormally high in animal fats and yet seemed to be immune to heart attacks as long as they did not move out of the community. A little more food for thought.

For those with a little more classical medical bent of mind one should mention the existence of the gerbil, a tiny Mongolian rodent who despite a fat-rich diet and levels of blood cholesterol shows no tendency toward atherosclerosis.

A number of other, similar findings exist and several more of these will be mentioned when the explanation for all this is elucidated.

Chapter 7

The Answer—Chlorine!

I have so far explained how heart attacks and strokes as well as certain other disorders are due to an underlying disease process called "atherosclerosis" wherein fatty materials are deposited in the inner lining of arteries, plugging them up. I presented the cholesterol theory of atherogenesis (atherosclerosis being related to high blood levels of cholesterol possibly other fats which in turn are contributed to by high dietary intake of cholesterol and "saturated" fats) only to reveal convincing evidence that this is not the whole answer. If the cholesterol theory is not the real answer, then one cannot protect oneself against heart attacks and strokes by avoiding dietary intake of cholesterol and other ("saturated") fats?

This is correct. I am not saying that cholesterol has no role whatsoever in atherogenesis and that therefore dietary habits make no difference at all. Cholesterol may be one of many contributing factors influencing atherogenesis and therefore dietary change may possibly affect the disease process to at least a small degree, just as other "risk factors" such as cigarette smoking, physical exercise, etc. may also have some influence on the matter. I am implying that even if a person changes his diet to one low in cholesterol and "saturated" fats, he is not guaranteeing himself immunity against heart attack and stroke. Persons who do not smoke get heart attacks and strokes (although admittedly less frequently than those who do.) The same statement is true for those who exercise regularly. And I am saying that the same is also true for persons who would change their dietary habits.

By now I should imagine that you, the reader, have become a little uneasy. I have told you that heart attacks and most strokes are the end result of a disease process called atherosclerosis, wherein the body's arteries are clogged up by fatty deposits (and the body's reaction to same) on their insides blocking the flow of blood to lesser or greater extent. I went on to present the classical, almost universally-accepted, cholesterol theory of atherogenesis including the alleged possibility of retarding the disease process by changing one's diet, especially with regards to intake of dietary fats. But then I proceeded to produce some intriguing ("anecdotal", the proponents of the cholesterol theory would allege) evidence which would not only tend to discredit this orthodox cholesterol theory, but also destroy the one ray of hope with regards to prevention of the disease process by means of dietary manipulation. You are probably wondering where do we go from here.

Fortunately, this book was not written merely to discredit the cholesterol theory and leave you (and everybody else) just hanging, "twisting slowly in the wind." [In the years since my original edition was written and published, several medically-lay authors have written quite interesting full-length books pointing out with many undeniable facts to back them up that atherosclerosis simply cannot be the result of eating normal foods containing natural cholesterol and "saturated" fats. But they cannot offer any alternate explanation to tell you how to keep from developing atherosclerosis and resultant heart attacks and strokes.] Have I, a practicing rural family doctor with no connections to any university medical research center, come up with an original theory that all the best medical minds in the entire world have overlooked over a period of many decades, with million and millions of unnecessary deaths from heart attack and stroke occurring in the meantime?

Indeed, I have.

And I have produced irrefutable scientific proofs of my unique Chlorine Theory, reproducible by anyone of average intelligence, to back up my revolutionary claims.

In retrospect, it is amazing how many separate observations point to the definitive solution of the problem of atherosclerosis and its consequences, mainly the common "heart attack" and most strokes, and yet have been ignored for almost a full century. It is truly a tragedy of historic proportions that modern, 20th Century medical science in its desperation to "look good" has grasped onto the almost childish cholesterol theory (even to the point of ignoring and denying absolutely proven facts which would tend to discredit this very simplistic theory) to the exclusion of all other possibilities. [The medical and medical research professions seem to be able in a remarkable way to consistently either ignore or else painfully twist all facts that do not conform to their preconceived notions of the cholesterol theory to fit their particular mold of what they think should be the truth. Therefore the classical cholesterol hypothesis (although I fairly consistently use the term "cholesterol theory in this publication, it actually does not meet the criteria of such word—it is truly merely a "hypothesis" by dictionary definition) essentially meets the explication of the concept of typical "mass delusion." It is just inconceivable to most medical men that such incredibly important, widespread, and basically untreatable disease as heart attack and stroke could have been essentially unknown less than a century ago. If this is true (as it is), it would mean that something has changed in the last 8 or 9 decades of human history but medical science has failed to "see the light." In all fairness, let me say the reasons for the amazing shortsightedness will seem to be a bit more understandable (although not truly justified) when it is realized what the culprit is and the initial circumstances of its widespread use.

As implied in the above paragraph, the great stumbling block which has inhibited rational, productive thinking about atherosclerosis was the unreasoning acceptance of the concept of the atheromatous diseases as being as old as mankind itself. Instead, as pointed out in previous chapters of this book, the atheromatous diseases, primarily heart attacks and most strokes, are not only less than a century old, but even today are almost entirely confined to populations under the influence of modern Western Civilization. So therefore we just look for some unique consideration of modern Western Civilization as the specific cause of these relatively new disease processes.

The first thing that always seems to be brought up today to separate our way of life from that of our ancestors in the past is an ill-defined entity called "stress." It is a fact that entire books have been written on this subject alone. Although I know it will bring cries of distress from certain quarters, let me dismiss this concept with regards to the present subject summarily by saying that if you think that you are living under stressful conditions today, what about the pioneer who had to keep his gun with him at all times in anticipation of unexpected Indian attack? He might have died from an arrow through his chest, but he never died of a heart attack! In those days a man walked the earth as a man until his dying days, not merely existing as a senile vegetable for years with the arteries to his brain clogged up as so many of our older people do today—of no use to themselves or anyone else and oftentimes a great burden, indeed, to their loved ones. Lest anyone try to discredit the above statement by saying, "But the life-expectancy back then was only 40 years and no one lived long enough to develop the modern "degenerative diseases", let us once again consider those sometimes uncomfortable things called "facts." The great increase in life-expectancy in the United States during the last century is mainly related to greatly decreased infant and childhood mortality! The cold, revealing figures show that if you are 50 years old right now your total life-expectancy is only a few months more than you great-grandfather's when he was 50 years old in 1900! There have always been considerable numbers of truly old people alive at any time in history, and in all countries of the world at that.

Next, we should consider the possibility of a deficit of some essential substance in the body. It seems most unlikely that there would be a nutritional deficit responsible for widespread grossly-evident diseases confined just to areas under the influence of modern Western Civilization. Quite the opposite would be more logical.

Finally, one is obligated to consider the possibility of the presence of foreign substances or the presence of abnormally large quantities of otherwise harmless materials in the body as a cause of disease. (This would basically be a matter of "poisoning.") The cholesterol theory of atherogenesis would fall under this category—the concept being that the presence of abnormally large quantities of fats derived from dietary intake are responsible for the disease processes. I (and several other authors of more recent books) have already debunked this nauseatingly simplistic hypothesis, despite the fact that it is one of the main "mass delusions" of both professionals and medically lay people of our age. But what about the validity of the above general idea of "poisoning" as applied to other substances?

We are living in an era unique in human history in many ways. But what is especially important is that each and every year many dozens of totally new chemical compounds are being introduced into our environment and consequently and inevitably into our bodies. The bodies of men throughout the history of human existence have been exposed to chemicals in the environment (mainly from foodstuffs, but also in some cases from pollution of air or water) which were not needed at best and possibly severely damaging—actually poisons. But throughout the millennia through the general processes of adaptation by means of survival of the fit (or those with fortunate genetics, etc.) the bodies of men have developed enzyme systems to handle most common natural poisons, at least to some really significant degree. Such adaptations of men and animals in general probably take countless hundreds of centuries. But as mentioned above, in the last several decades chemicals totally alien to living organisms (many of which must be frankly considered to be poisons) have been and are at present being introduced in an incredibly increasing number of forms and amounts. Therefore when one is studying disease entities which are of very recent origin (e.g. the atheromatous diseases, less than a century old) one must give prime consideration to the possibility of such diseases being the result of poisoning—a reaction to a chemical new to the species and to which it has not had the time or ability to adapt.

If heart attacks and strokes are indeed due to a form of insidious, chronic poisoning, to where are we to look for the source? There are only a few ways in which chemical substances, including those which must be classified as exogenous poisons, can enter the body. They are: directly through the skin, via the air we breathe into our lungs, or via substances ingested into the alimentary tract, ie. food or liquids such as water.

Trying to discern the exact substances which may be involved in a form of poisoning involves truly a myriad of possibilities, and it is easy to become confused and misled. But as alluded to above, there have been made certain observations of extreme importance, which point the way to the ultimate truth. Others have ignored or denied the importance or even the genuine existence of these findings because they lead away from the generally accepted hypotheses or theories. It is sad that we are in an era of "group think" and procedure by committee. As a great educator once put it, "Could 'Hamlet' have been written by a committee? Creative ideas—spring from individuals." [Today, if the research "peer review" committee doesn't approve, it isn't going anywhere, fast; the truly creative individual learns this lesson the hard way early in his career and usually turns his energies to making money where one's rewards are immediate and evident to all. Society as a whole loses really big, but it never realizes the facts related to that saddest of all plaintive phrases, "What could have been."]

Just what are these all-important observations and to what do they point? Because the author of this publication believes that it may be of some future interest to medical historians, the original observation which led to this amazing new theory of atherogenesis about to be expounded will be singled out and mentioned first. [This breakthrough discovery involves a leap of the imagination, and anything originating or derived in such a manner is pure anathema to the medical and medical research establishment. The absolute validity of similar future *in vitro* experiments as regards to extrapolation to living systems is of little importance. What was important is that it provided the nidus for a whole new stream of thought.

This was the seemingly insignificant and widely known fact that in the dairy industry very tenacious, yellowish deposits build up on milk utensils washed in certain kinds of germicide solutions. It was evident that some chemical in the water used to wash the utensils reacted with milk or some component of milk to produce a deposit. The biological analogy should be obvious.

Have there been any experiments reported in the medical literature relating water and elements contained therein to coronary heart disease? It has been shown most convincingly that the harder (higher concentrations of ionized inorganic minerals) the drinking water, the less the incidence of coronary heart disease; and that the hardness of the drinking water is related to no other known diseases except heart and vascular disease.

By now, I assume that the reader will have taken the not-too-subtle hints (like the title of this chapter!) and come to the conclusion that there must be something in the drinking water that is the culprit. And in one short, succinct sentence I am making the point that the *specific cause of atherosclerosis and resulting heart attacks and most strokes is none other than the ubiquitous CHLORINE purposely added as a disinfectant to all "treated" drinking water!!!*

It is, in my opinion, certainly one of the greatest paradoxes of recorded history that one of the very same public health measures which has been primarily responsible for the great increases in statistical life expectancy in the Western world should also, unsuspectedly, be specifically responsible for the most important chronic diseases of later life.

It should now be manifestly apparent why no medical scientist has ever even for a fleeting moment entertained the truth in this matter. Chlorine is a classical "sacred cow" of modern medical science. Is it conceivable that something of such obvious and wonderful utility, so widely used, and with no apparent acute side effects could be responsible for all heart attacks and most strokes, the main disease scourges of modern times? Is it not incredibly difficult to believe that millions upon millions of dollars and incalculable hours of time have been poured down the drain by thousands of well-paid medical researchers busily and eruditely engaged in finding answers to the wrong questions? And although the two chemicals are totally unrelated, anyone opposing the use of chlorine would be immediately disregarded as an antifluoridation-type "nut." What medical scientist/researcher would risk tarnishing his reputation and grant-collecting future by espousing a theory which would automatically be tainted in the popular mind due to the confusion between the terms, "chlorine" versus "fluoride", as well as lack of distinction in the popular, medically-lay mind between "chlorine" and "chloride."

This is, it may be recalled, not the first time in modern medical history that a presumably innocuous chemical substance has been indicted as an agent of serious disease. Some years ago blindness caused by a disease known as retrolental fibroplasia was distressingly common among children born prematurely. Only some years after this form of blindness had become distressingly prevalent was it discovered that it was being caused by high concentrations of life-supporting oxygen in incubators. [Thereafter this form of blindness was virtually unknown until the fairly recent advent of great advances in the pediatric subspecialty of neonatology resulted in the saving of very small and very sick premature infants. The presumably necessary use of oxygen in such situations now causes about as many cases of blindness as occurred in the 1940s.]

You will, of course, now want to know on what basis can I make the sweeping statement that chlorine in "treated" drinking water is the greatest crippler and killer of modern times, ie. the prime causative agent of atherosclerosis and its killer clinical syndromes, the common heart attack (also known as "coronary thrombosis" and "myocardial infarction" or "MI") and the great majority of strokes [now being called "brain attack" in some medical circles.]

Let us retrace out steps and see if my new Chlorine Theory of atherogenesis will explain satisfactorily the same facts I used to disparage the classical and universally accepted cholesterol hypothesis:

Great emphasis was put previously on the concept that the heart attack was an essentially unknown entity before about 1920 and did not become of sufficient significance to affect mortality statistics until about 1930. How do these facts correlate with the use of elemental chlorine in "treated" drinking water? The answer is that experimental use of chlorine to "purify" city water supplies did not begin until the late 1890s. Chlorination gained relatively wide acceptance in the second decade of the 20th century and in the third decade (1920s) it was found that satisfactory killing of organisms was dependent upon a residual concentration of chlorine in the water at point of use above the amount necessary to react chemically with organic impurities. When it is remembered that evidence of clinical disease takes at least 10 to 20 years to develop, it becomes evident that there is a close correlation between the introduction of widespread chlorination of water supplies and the origin and increasing incidence of heart attacks that is exceedingly difficult to explain away.

In light of the Chlorine Theory just presented, we can now understand why there were no heart attacks in England during the 19th century despite a significant portion of the population consuming diets very high in saturated animal fats. We can understand why the Eskimos, whose diet was composed in the majority of animal fats, used to be immune to coronary heart attacks and other manifestations of atherosclerosis. Why heart attacks have been totally unknown among the Chinese until recent decades and still are basically unknown among Chinese farm workers. Why most primitive peoples, and to this day most sub-Saharan black people in Africa, don't have to worry about having a heart attack. Why the residents of Roseto, Pennsylvania had no heart attacks unless they moved to another community. And why American zoo animals are starting to show atherosclerosis, something totally unknown in the wild.

There was no chlorinated drinking water in England during the 19th century. Eskimos in the past may have consumed huge quantities of dietary fats, but their drinking water was pure, melted snow. Chlorine in the drinking water was and is unknown among primitive peoples, and until recently in most parts of sub-Saharan Africa. The Chinese have been thought of in the past by some as a poor people who spread their sewage on the ground and got worms in their guts from drinking contaminated water and eating filthy food. We in the Western world are more civilized—we take our sewage and dump it into our rivers. We then drain the same dilute sewage into our water supplies, filter it, and inject chlorine into it. We don't get worms in our guts from the water, but we sure do get something else! The inhabitants of Roseto drank water straight from flowing mountain streams, but when they moved to the big city and drank chlorinated water like all the other city dwellers they were subject to the same retribution. [God and nature are not respecters of persons; break the rules and you will suffer the consequences.] The animals in our American zoos are being given chlorinated city water and as should be expected, are starting to develop atherosclerosis.

Although not mentioned before, the Japanese who normally have had a very low rate of heart attacks are no different from other people when they move to Hawaii—and drink chlorinated water. The Masai tribesmen of Kenya have almost no heart disease although they eat at least as much cholesterol as most Americans—but drink no chlorinated water. Coronary heart disease was unknown among a group of 500 poor Irish farm workers studied by famed Dr. Paul Dudley White while being widespread among their chlorine-drinking brothers in the United States. And, contrary to popular belief, high level business executives (supposedly under much chronic stress) have a statistically lower incidence of heart attacks than their subordinates. (In America, when an executive reaches the highest echelons not only does he receive a key to his own "washroom", but while at the office drinks non-chlorinated bottled water.) The lowly gerbil drinks no water at all, instead manufacturing all the water it needs from the dry food it eats, and therefore escapes the end results of chronic chlorine poisoning.

We can understand even the intriguing, apparently unrelated and sometimes apparently facetious facts and correlations presented before. The documented lower incidence of coronary heart disease in areas with hard water could possibly be explained by postulating chemical reactions between the free chlorine, an extremely active chemical substance, and the ions which cause hardness of water resulting in biologically innocuous chlorides. (This suggestion is not to exclude the possibility of some other, more complex biological mode of action of the hard water ions.) Even the strange and apparently facetious correlations between the number of telephones per unit of population and the cardiac death rate can be explained on the basis that chlorinated drinking water and telephones are both products of modern civilization, both became widespread in the early decades of the last century, and both are most prevalent in urbanized areas.

[This telephones and cardiac death rate comparison should serve as a good example of the common error of presuming that if events occur temporally together such correlation by itself implies a true causative relationship. Beware the usual tendency to imply a causative relationship simply on the basis of mere correlation of events or findings.]

There is one other very important situation that we should not forget to mention. During the Korean War autopsies were performed on otherwise apparently healthy soldiers killed in battle. In articles in the Journal of the American Medical Association [Enos, W.F.; Holmes, R.H.; Beyer, J.C. "Coronary Disease Among U.S. Soldiers Killed in Action in Korea" JAMA 152: 1090-1093, 1953. Enos, W.F.; Beyer, J.C.; Holmes, R.H. "Pathogenesis of Coronary Disease in American Soldiers Killed in Korea" JAMA 158: 912-914, 1955.] it was reported that among the soldiers whose average age at death was 22.1 years, over 75% showed some gross evidence of coronary arteriosclerosis. These results have been widely discussed over the years with the usual conclusion being that coronary artery disease is far more common and extensive than previously suspected, especially in young men. In light of my new Chlorine Theory I most strongly question this interpretation and conclusion. If you ask any man who served in that war, he will tell you that the water for our soldiers in Korea was so heavily chlorinated that it was almost undrinkable. And the comparable incidence of coronary artery disease in men of the same age in civilian life was well known from routine autopsy statistics to be far less than that found in their contemporaries killed in action in Korea. Incidentally, discussions I had with Korean physicians revealed that heart attacks were almost totally unknown among their fellow countrymen. Koreans in their native land for the most part drink un-"purified" water.

More recent similar postmortem studies performed on U.S. casualties in Vietnam have shown an even higher incidence of coronary disease. Being a miserably hot country, the average GI cold not avoid drinking large quantities of incredibly highly chlorinated water. The water made available for soldiers in Vietnam was required to contain a minimum of 5 ppm (parts per million) of residual chlorine. But I can tell you from personal experience (in the infantry in Vietnam during the worst of the war) that because only a minimum standard was required by regulations, oftentimes the water was chlorinated at a level several times that—levels quite comparable to those in my animal experiments to be described! "Results" of drinking hyperchlorinated water on the unsuspecting soldiers seems to be exactly the same as on the animals in my experiments. Apparently there is a straight-line direct causal relationship/correlation between the amount of chlorine ingested and the speed and degree of development of atherosclerosis!

It is very interesting that clinical material (specimens obtained at operation or autopsy) has shown atherosclerosis in synthetic vascular grafts (artificial Dacron fabric arteries) in human beings. One cannot help but think of the analogy between this and the deposition of "milkstone" on smooth rubber or metal surfaces. In both we have the flow of fat and cholesterol-containing fluids over surfaces in the presence of free chlorine, with resultant surface deposits. If this analogy would hold true (who knows?), it would be powerful evidence in favor of the so-called "encrustation" theory of the mechanics of atheroma formation, the main differences seen in the artery lining being due to the body's reaction to the deposit. One should note that the encrustation theory offered no explanation for the basic etiology of atherosclerosis. All it did was try to explain how the deposit formed in a physical sense, not why it formed.

Some of the previous examples suggest strongly that dietary consumption of fats bears but little relationship to the development of atherosclerosis. This is not to say, however, that there is absolutely no connection whatsoever between dietary fats, hypercholesterolemia (high blood cholesterol levels) and atherogenesis. To avoid later misinterpretation, let me emphasize that atherogenesis involves a system of multiple factors in its etiology. This is to say that factors such as diet under some circumstances, exercise, smoking habits, etc. may be of some significance—at least possibly related to the speed of development of atherosclerosis under the condition of exposure to exogenous elemental chlorine from drinking water.

In any system of multiple etiology, the primary agent (in atherosclerosis the primary agent is chlorine) is only one cause in the overall expression of the disease. But it must be an essential cause. For example, it would be inconceivable for tuberculosis to occur in the absence of the tubercle bacillus. Nevertheless it is recognized that there are multiple other causes or influences than the primary agent (the tubercle bacillus in this example) in the production of clinical tuberculosis disease. Thus the primary agent must be an essential cause (the disease of tuberculosis cannot occur under any circumstances whatsoever in the absence of the germ) though not necessarily a sufficient cause (clinical tuberculosis may not occur even in the presence of the bacillus, e.g. positive tuberculin skin reaction in a clinically healthy person.) Likewise, in the process of atherogenesis, chlorine is the essential agent (under the vast majority of circumstances atherosclerosis cannot occur to a clinically significant degree, ie. severe enough to cause manifestations such as heart attack or stroke, in the absence of chlorine regardless of diet or other contributing factors, though it is not necessarily a sufficient cause (e.g. normally healthy menstruating women never develop atherosclerosis or it complications even if they are exposed to chlorine and the other factors.)

Chapter 8

Medical Research In The U.S.—A Racket?

No radical and new theory, especially one of the immediate and practical importance of that presented in this book, is complete without at least some preliminary and, presumably, convincing experimental proofs. But before we immerse ourselves in this somewhat technical aspect, let me air a most distressing situation which has permeated the very guts of American scientific endeavor. Our universities and medical schools are thoroughly infiltrated with professional research parasites who are interested in only a few things—mainly money, prestige, and fat retirement checks, all paid by the taxpayer. Basic medical research has been elevated to the status of a demigod in America. And make no mistake, as a result of this it has entered the realm of financial big business, with all the inherent potential immorality and evilness of same. Basic medical research is big business in terms of yearly monetary expenditures—millions upon millions of dollars are spent each year by what amounts to essentially a university monopoly, run by firmly- entrenched, self-designated "research specialists." And what have been the results? In 1966, for example, the National Cancer Institute had spent about $500 million (that's right, half-a-billion dollars) in testing just 170 drugs without any results applicable to the common types of cancers. [This situation in general has become far, far worse since the first edition of this book was written.] It makes one wonder if these researchers really do want to find a cure for cancer, or anything else. Or are they just primarily concerned with perpetuating their neverending gravy train. And this type of situation is the rule rather than the exception!

What is wrong? It really boils down to another example of the possibility of big money and prestige corrupting absolutely. Make no mistake, I am not condemning medical research *per se* by any means, but rather what has happened to much medical research in America in present times. No longer does a scientist think out a possible solution to a problem and then go to the laboratory to obtain proof supporting his hypothesis. Today with all kinds of monies available, the prestige and money-hungry researchers (and by implication, the prestige and money-hungry universities and medical schools) obtain financial grants and then go directly to the laboratory hoping that lightning will strike from heaven above and they will "happen" upon some finding of scientific interest, or, miracle of miracles, even something of scientific importance!

Certain university medical centers have realized the extent of their involvement in this financial big-business to the point where they have hired full-time public relations men to tout their researchers. Witness the rash of extravagant and unwarranted claims concerning organ (e.g. heart) transplants! A good PR man can be worth millions of dollars each and every year to an "prestigious" medical research center.

[In the present medical/medically-related field the best research in the last few decades is being done by scientists employed by the pharmaceutical firms. These firms are out to make a profit, and these employees have to produce, not just publish meaningless "scientific", "peer-reviewed" journal articles. I just can't tell you how many marvelous new drugs/medications have been introduced during the last 30 or so years. You will note that the government/government researchers have almost no (otherwise than oftentimes impeding regulatory) role in the development of these remarkable and oftentimes absolutely marvelous medicines or their introduction. Clinical research, the hands-on development and use of surgical procedures, use of medicines, medical devices and machines and so on has also yielded incredibly wonderful, life-saving and life-prolonging advances. The real bummer has been the results of the so-called "basic" research conducted at big universities, and government and so-called "independent" research institutes, invariably taxpayer supported. They can (and do) spread their propaganda about the necessity of "basic" research (in medical or other fields) but the truth of the matter is that there are two overwhelming problems involved with such. First of all, without any specific goals in mind no one in any field of endeavor (or in life itself, for that matter) can accomplish anything much of value. Accomplishments result from pursuing goals, not spending 90+% of your time obtaining funding and then hoping to stumble over something. As important as this above first matter may be, the other consideration is that these "basic research" setups represent almost pure socialism, a system that is at its roots satanic, truly evil. Friend, if "the path to hell is paved with good intentions", the absolutely best example of this is socialism! Any socialistic endeavor, including specifically government (taxpayer)-funded research, medical or otherwise, is very poorly or totally non-productive because of the underlying fact that useful, productive endeavor in any type of socialistic setup is unrewarded. Sloth and lack of useful results are inevitably excused and not punished in such a system. ("Basic' research isn't supposed to produce useful results", say the "scientific" apologists.) Inevitably, and no matter how well-intentioned initially, the members/employees of a socialistic endeavor assuredly and without exception become parasitic bureaucrats with the only goal that of tenure, preserving their employment until they can retire on a fat pension.

Chapter 9

The Experimental Proof Of The Cholesterol Theory

In contrast to the situation just mentioned, the proofs about to be offered are scientific experiments purposefully planned to offer direct and straightforward support to or refutation of a previously well thought-out theory.

While it should be understood that the results of animal experiments cannot ever be extrapolated directly to apply to human beings without the ever-present risk of error due to inherent biological differences (human beings are not dogs or rabbits or chickens—remember that the drug Thalidomide was "proven" to be free from deformity causing side effects by experiments with dogs), there are many instances where if due attention is given to possible sources of error the final conclusions may be quite real and useful. As can be readily realized, there are many important medical experiments which cannot ever be performed on human subjects, at least in a society where we do give at least lip-service to the concept of inherent worth of human beings and human dignity. Thus we must turn to animal experimentation on a regular basis.

Significant atherosclerosis is almost totally unknown among wild animals, just as it is among primitive peoples. Under special circumstances, however, animals of certain species have been made to develop at least some of the early plaques of atherosclerosis in their arteries. With rabbits it is necessary to give the experimental bunnies diets high in added cholesterol (quite obviously a grossly abnormal situation for a normally vegetarian animal.) To use the dog, a diet high in cholesterol will not do, by itself. In order to induce atherosclerosis in the canine species, it is necessary to destroy the animals' thyroid glands either by surgical removal or by administration of radioactive iodine.

The one other animal species extensively used in the experimental production of atherosclerosis is the lowly chicken. Some researchers claim that the chicken is prone to spontaneous development of lesions of atherosclerosis, ie., even when given an apparently normal diet. As will soon be shown, this is not true at all. Nevertheless, the chicken has been shown to be an excellent experimental animal species for the purpose at hand. (Indeed, it has been widely accepted that the chicken is as good as or better than any other animal for research in atherosclerosis in procedures designed to help analyze pathogenesis and/or therapeutic value of different regimens and substances.)

With this knowledge in mind, the author set up a controlled experimental situation using the chicken as the experimental species.

There were two general phases to the experimental proof of my Chlorine Theory. In the first, 100 day-old cockerels were divided into two groups of 50 each. With the understanding in mind that what was to be proven or disproven was that chlorine is the essential (though not necessarily sufficient) cause of atherosclerosis, the two groups were set up with known contributory causes acting on both, the only difference being the presence of chlorine—the presumed essential cause—in the drinking water and mash (food) of the experimental group and absent from the food and water of the controls.

The male of the species was chosen in the knowledge that just like in human beings it is the male which is primarily susceptible to the development of atherosclerosis. (All other experiments regarding atherosclerosis using the chicken species which have been reported in the medical literature have used cockerels for the same reason.)

Both groups were placed on a cooked mash consisting of about a 1:1 mixture of corn and oat meals with about 5% low-priced oleomargarine added. Pure distilled water was used exclusively. Chlorine was added to the drinking water and mash of the experimental group in the form of chlorine bleach (hypochlorite disinfectant), about one-third teaspoonful per quart of water. This very highly chlorinated water (purposefully highly chlorinated, as the cause/effect response was thought to probably be a linear one) was first given to the experimental group at twelve weeks of age.

The results were nothing short of spectacular! Within three weeks there were grossly observable effects on both appearance and behavior. The experimental group became lethargic, huddling in corners except at feeding time. Their feathers became frayed and dirty and these cockerels walked around with their wings hunched up, their feathers fluffed up like they were always cold (the experiment was performed in an unheated barn in winter), their pale combs drooping. This appearance is most suggestive of symptoms resulting from clogging up of the micro-circulation.

Meanwhile the control group was the epitome of vigorous health. They were much larger in size than the experimental group, active, quarrelsome, vigorous-appearing with smooth, clean, shiny feathers and bright combs held up erectly.

No less remarkable was the gross appearance of the aortas, or main blood vessels. The abdominal aorta (the place where atherosclerosis is known to occur in chickens) of all the cockerels dying after four months were carefully examined. In more than 95% of the experimental group grossly visible thick yellow plaques of typical atherosclerosis protruding into lumens were discovered! This group of chickens was noted to have an extremely high apparently spontaneous death rate and common findings on examination of the carcasses were hemorrhage into the lungs and enlarged hearts. Although no blood pressure readings were taken during the experiment, these findings are suggestive of gross arterial hypertension.

At seven months there were so few experimental group chickens remaining alive that the survivors were sacrificed, with identical findings upon necropsy. At the same time one-third of the apparently healthy control group was also sacrificed with not one abnormal aorta found!

Although these results seemed conclusive, it was decided to repeat the procedures by taking the remaining healthy control animals of the first experiment and dividing them also into an experimental group receiving chlorine and a continuing control group. Once again the roosters receiving chlorine showed fantastic gross changes in appearance and behavior within three weeks. The first change noted was a remarkable paleness of the combs. Instead of bright fiery red the combs became nearly orange in color and soon began to droop. These changes were shortly followed by the ones described for the original experimental group and, as expected, gross atheromas of the aortas were found on examination within three months of the commencement of this part of the experiment.

To summarize, in both experimental groups gross changes in appearance and behavior, most likely explicable by postulating obstruction of the micro-circulation, were evident within a few weeks in the fowls receiving chlorine. These changes were followed by development of gross atherosclerotic lesions of the aortas evident within a couple of months. Control groups treated in an identical manner except for the absence of added chlorine remained healthy and vigorous, grew well, and showed no evidence of either atherosclerosis of the aorta or symptoms of possible obstruction of the micro-circulation. [After all these years I'll admit that, not to be wasteful, my father and I butchered the remaining control group roosters and ate them. They were delicious!]

As a related comment, it should be mentioned that the so-called "spontaneous avian (chicken) atherosclerosis" reported in the medical literature was not spontaneous at all. These experiments, as well as most others on dogs and rabbits, were performed in urban university canters using city water which inadvertently contained chlorine. Chickens raised on farms with well water but never show any signs of atherosclerosis. A related fact is that it has been noted that animals in our zoos are starting to show evidence of atherosclerosis. Once again, the culprit is the ubiquitous chlorinated city water.

Chapter 10

Practical Suggestions

About now the reader of this book is getting more than a little concerned about the water he has been drinking and will drink in the future. Go to the water tap and draw yourself a big glass of water. Now hold it up and look at it. What does it mean to you? Perhaps by now you are a little angry—it is the insidious poison contained in that very glass of water which has been responsible for so much suffering and death of the last century. Undoubtedly you know men (and women) who have been cut down in the prime of life by heart attacks or strokes. Friends, probably close relatives, and maybe even you have had problems, yourself! More men have died from heart attacks during the last two years in the United States alone than have been killed in all of our many wars since our country was founded. And have you ever seen an active, vitally alive human being reduced to a state little more than that of an inanimate vegetable by a stroke?

But rather than being upset, you should be overjoyed. Soon the coronary heart attack and stroke should be no more—mere uneasy memories of a blind and ignorant past. Ever since the conquering of infectious diseases earlier in this century by the intelligent use of public health measures (primarily sanitation) and in more recent years by the use of antibiotic medicines, the chronic diseases of the aging population have come to the fore. But now two of the most important "degenerative" disease have been conquered. Now our American citizens may truly enjoy the joys of "life in the years" instead of mere years in their lives.

[In the first edition of this book I was incredibly naive enough to hope that the wonderful message contained therein would be readily accepted, at least by medically lay persons, that our municipal water treatment plants would be converted with all due speed to provide clean, chlorine-free water, and the problems of heart attacks (and most strokes) would be solved. Only after twenty years has someone (The Nader Report) besides me even proposed a change in the way municipal water supplies are treated, without the use of chlorine—such chlorine now known to produce carcinogens (cancer-causing agents) from the already highly contaminated raw water (as well as atherosclerosis/heart attack/ stroke as described in this book.) In view of the fact that it may take another twenty years before anything at all changes with regards to municipal water treatment on a large scale, what can a person do here and now to protect himself from the ravages of chlorine? At the time I wrote the original edition of this book the choices were limited, indeed. Few people had good deep well water available. "Spring mineral" water was a good option, presuming no chlorine was added. Commercially distilled water was another option. But thirty years ago the home water purification device industry was in its infancy, and chlorine was a "sacred cow" to the great majority of health professionals and consequently the general population. I am proud of the fact that the first edition of this book changed this important (and growing more important with the passing of each day) industry. Not only are many, many more personal/home water purification devices/options available, but I find it personally very interesting that almost every ad or piece of promotional literature states first that the produce "removes chlorine", and many quote me directly from the first edition of this book. Chlorine in drinking water is not any longer the "sacred cow" that it used to be, with ordinary Americans not knowledgeable about this book and my Chlorine Theory still vaguely aware of something "wrong" regarding such.

The situation regarding possible practical solutions to the problem of chlorine in drinking water has changed radically since the publication of the first edition of this book. Bottled water has become a big, big industry. Most bottled soft drinks and fruit juice drinks are made with "filtered" water. Use of untreated deep well water, bottled or "spring water", "deionized" water, and distilled water remain very viable options. But the biggest change over the years has been the introduction of personal and house water purification devices and systems to remove chlorine, as well as other contaminants. The cheapest and simplest device for the home or other "point of use" is the activated carbon/charcoal water filter in its various and sundry forms, types and permutations now available. The filters include many various types, small, big, flow-through, countertop, below counter, silver impregnated, plain activated carbon, cheap, expensive, and so forth. (It may be strange to say so, but I find it remarkable, in my mind, almost preordained, that a rather readily available and relatively cheap substance, activated carbon/charcoal is so incredibly efficient in removing dangerous chlorine from drinking water. It is almost as if God provided a remarkable answer before the problem ever became manifest.) As a practical matter, it should be noted that activated charcoal filters should always be used with cold water as they do not work well with hot water. Other alternative home water treatments include the "high tech" (and expensive) systems which use the "reverse osmosis" principle, after the water has been put through a more conventional activated carbon filter, which clean out many more other contaminants than a simple filter. I believe that a personal system using ultraviolet light rays for killing bacteria rather than chlorine has been introduced. Devices using ozone to kill harmful organisms are another alternative. And, finally, there are home distillation units available, still very much a viable alternative if a bit expensive to operate.

There are those who claim that chlorine can be absorbed into the body through the intact skin (or via breathing it into the lungs?) during showers and baths. I have obtained no specific data on this situation, but personally I have always avoided chlorinated water completely, even for showers! There have been marketed devices to attach to a shower head to adsorb the chlorine from the water as it flows through it, and if I had to regularly take showers with chlorinated water I would most certainly buy such a device and use it. "Better safe than sorry."

In the last thirty years or so there has been noted a significant drop in the incidence of heart attacks in the United States. Orthodox medicine cannot come up with a reasonable explanation for this phenomena. May I suggest that such relative drop in heart attacks is specifically due to less individual ingestion of chlorine by Americans. There has been a massive change in Americans' drinking (water, not booze) habits over the past 30 years. To put it plainly, a majority of Americans do not regularly drink chlorinated tap water anymore! (No, I am not going to claim specific responsibility for this change in Americans' habits, despite its laudatory effects with regards to reducing total chlorine consumption.) In the recent relatively good economic times Americans have turned en masse to drinking bottled water and soft drinks. Many almost never go to the water tap for a drink anymore! (The stereotype of younger Americans with a bottle of cola in their hand or within reach at almost all times has a definite basis in reality.) And I think that from a demographic point of view this unrecognized change, resulting in significantly decreased chlorine ingestion, has been so massive in its nature to actually have reduced the prevalence of atherosclerosis and heart attacks!

A problem for which I have no good (or at least cheap) answer at this time relates to the fact that the U.S. Environmental Protection Agency has for some years now been forcing American city water treatment plants to change from pure chlorination to use of a combination of chlorine and ammonia (chloramines). While this action is supposed to reduce the production of chlorine complexes (chlorinated organic materials) to reduce the incidence of (relatively very rare) bladder cancer allegedly caused by the use of chlorine alone, it has opened a whole new "bag of worms." Specifically, the usual activated carbon/charcoal water filters can be somewhat inefficient in taking these chlorine-ammonia compounds out of the water. In addition, while ordinary chlorinated tap water will evaporate the chlorine out into the air by simply standing at room temperatures, such does not happen with these relatively new chlorine-ammonia compounds. Undoubtedly, the expensive "reverse osmosis" devices will work, but it is more than a bit upsetting that the EPA has forced the water treatment plants to purposefully put "something" into the water that cannot be effectively removed by usual means. A great irony of this matter is that the U.S. government got us all into these problems of atherosclerosis and its sequelae starting early in the 20th century, by forcing the use of elemental chlorine on an emergency basis because of the then-raging typhoid epidemics. This was done without any tests or what would now be called "research" regarding possible chronic effects on human beings ingesting this powerful, extremely chemically-active material, chlorine. And now, going into the 21st Century, the EPA is forcing Americans to drink other frighteningly active chemicals—again with absolutely no prior tests regarding possible chronic effects! I know (and the whole purpose of this book is to let you know) that the elemental chlorine used for water "purification" is the specific cause of athero-sclerosis and its disease syndromes of heart attack and most strokes. But what these "chloramines" do in the human body, whether they are more or less dan-gerous than simple elemental chlorine, I simply do not know. The EPA has done some studies on the effects of these chloramines (see copy of letter at front of this book signed by Donald J. Ehreth), but they sure have not made the results public to date.

Getting back to "practical advice", when looking into buying a chlorine-removing device/system you will find that every manufacturer and salesman can give multiple reasons why their particular one is the very best. "Buyer beware", because in this as in most purchases you always have to pay for what you get (the "no free lunch" concept), but you may not always get what you pay for. But for the purposes of this book, if it takes out the chlorine it's worth it! Purified water and/or devices to purify water may not be cheap, but they are a heck of a lot cheaper than a heart attack or stroke. So make a real investment in your and your family's health, provide yourself and your household with chlorine-free water as soon as possible! If you plan on the government to do it, to protect you from harm, you will likely be waiting forever (or at least until you die of that heart attack.) Get yourself a source of chlorine-free drinking water now!!

While it is true that the development of atherosclerosis is a slow process in human beings under ordinary circumstances of exposure to chlorine in usual municipal water system residual concentrations, your personal clock to disaster has been ticking along for years. Only fools tempt fate. Why drink another sin-gle glass of that poisonous dilute sewage called tapwater? Chlorine-free water for drinking is as close as your local supermarket/grocery store. With the immediate problem solved in this manner you can then make rational choices regarding possible further action to ensure chlorine-free drinking water for the rest of your (longer) life. Continuing to buy chlorine-free bottled, distilled, deionized, or "spring water": indefinitely may be the perfect solution for you. Probably a greater number of concerned persons will eventually opt for the convenience of one of the activated carbon/charcoal filter systems, a really excellent choice with regards to the cost/benefit ration (specifically with regards to removal of chlorine, the point of this book.) Finally, there are those who are also concerned with the many hundreds of other contaminants possibly present in drinking water, and who have the financial resources to afford "top of the line" true "purification" devices that remove 90%+ of all contaminants, namely, properly vented water distillation setups and the latest development in the field, the technologically advanced reverse osmosis units with final activated carbon filtration.

Chapter 11

Is Existing Atherosclerosis Reversible?

[I have made no qualms regarding the fact that it is chlorine that is the specific cause (ie. essential, if not necessarily sufficient} cause of atherosclerosis. It follows that avoidance of ingestion of chlorine will prevent the further development of atherosclerosis and resultant heart attack/stroke/other atheromatous-based disease process.

The question that naturally follows is "Is existing atherosclerosis reversible?"

Thank heavens, the answer is a plain, straightforward "Yes, existing atherosclerosis is reversible!" The best demographic evidence that correlates with this claim is the fact that American Korean War and Vietnam War soldiers who were the "guinea pigs" in the inadvertent "ultimate proof" of the Chlorine Theory did not all die of heart attacks in the first few years after their return to the States and resumption of more usual levels of chlorine intake. In order to have ended up with no more than average atherosclerotic disease for their age group, the atherosclerotic clogging of their arteries must have actually regressed (become less) even though chlorine intake was continued, although at far lower levels than while in a fighting war zone. These facts also lend credence to my claim of the direct dose-response relationship between chlorine ingested and degree of development of atherosclerosis. It would appear, from the facts and explanation just elucidated, that not only is there a direct dose-response relationship between chlorine and atherosclerosis in the development of the disease processes, but that (at least under some circumstances, e.g. relatively young men with high-degree arterial blockage secondary to very high levels of chlorine intake under war situations) there will be apparently "spontaneous" decreases in the level of atherosclerotic involvement of the arteries merely by decreasing the dose of the chlorine!

Another very strong piece of evidence pointing to the likelihood of the reversibility of chlorine-caused atherosclerosis is the fact that autopsies of persons dying in a "cachectic" state, either from old-fashioned starvation (e.g. World War II) or of the "starvation" of metastatic cancer, show clear arteries. This is true even when the victims were positively known to have severe atherosclerosis prior to the development of the cachectic state, and, presumably even in the presence of continuing chlorine intake. (The "Pritikin diet" of years past may have worked at times, to at least some degree, for the exact same reason, ie., it is, if followed faithfully with its fat and caloric restrictions, actually a true "starvation" diet.)

In the meantime, it should be obvious that before considering the concept of the reversal of atherosclerosis, we must stop further development of the atherosclerotic clogging of our arteries. And that means complete and total avoidance of all chlorine in our drinking water! (And personally I have always avoided even showering in chlorinated water; some investigators have suggested the possibility of chlorine getting into the body directly through the skin.) The practical, here-and-now things are what should concern you at this point. Academic-type considerations of the probability of reversing existing atherosclerosis is meaningless if you are developing further arterial deposits by still drinking typical urban, chlorinated, dilute sewage cocktails! So, as just mentioned in the previous chapter, get off your duff and get some chlorine-free bottled/"Spring"/deionized/distilled water right now. Then later you can take your time to consider the number of choices available, e.g. to continue buying chlorine-free drinking water or investing in a water treatment/purification device.

Chapter 12

Insidious Chemical Poisoning And The Future

As I bring this book ["Part I" of this revised edition] to a close, may I end on a somewhat pessimistic, but honest, note. As mentioned in some detail before, our environment and truly the whole world is becoming increasingly contaminated with new chemicals, the ultimate effects on living organisms including man being almost totally unknown. Most of these substances are at least in some degree cumulative poisons. The ghastly effects of the drug Thalidomide in producing malformed children was overlooked, obvious thought it was in hindsight, for several years, ie. until it was obvious to anyone. The fantastic long-range effects of chlorine ingestion were not in the least even fleetingly suspected for more than two-thirds of a century. How many other potentially harmful chemical compounds are we being exposed to every day? A cursory glance at the labels in any supermarket is enough to make one shudder with horror. We worry about atomic fallout, but the chemical "fallout" in our environment may be of vastly greater significance over the long run to the human race. Alas, the chemical pollution of our environment is a very profitable business.

Chapter 13

The Author vs. The Establishment

In the form of a sort of postscript let me say that I fully expect to encounter vast quantities of hostility from professional ignorance and jealousy. [The statement has, unfortunately, been proven true innumerable times since it was penned more than thirty years ago.] In the best of times organized medicine has been known to oppose almost all revolutionary advances. This holds throughout history—witness the scorn heaped upon Drs. Simmelweiss and Holmes in the 19th century when they insisted that doctors themselves were spreading childbed fever by refusing to wash their filthy hands between checking patients. Or more recently the disgraceful resistance to the adoption of Sister Kenney's therapy for poliomyelitis (later adopted and expanded on greatly—and made "proper" by calling it "physical therapy", with now even a medical specialty of such called "physical medicine' or ":physiatry.") Sister Kenney was a mere nurse who did not spend hundreds of thousands of dollars "researching." And a history of the opposition to the use of anesthesia makes fascinating, if horrifying, reading. These are but a few examples of a long, embarrassing list. [A list to which my present saga will someday be added!]

I realize that in this book I have stepped on many feet. There is probably nothing more sacred to modern (university medical center) medicine than that mystical thing called "basic medical research", which I have debunked in part, at least the dishonest way in which much of it is now practiced. The potential damage from this is more than just related to a matter of principle—a lot of very influential persons in many important places and positions are dependent financially on taxpayer-supplied medical research funds. Eventually, inadvertently some will suffer from a monetary standpoint from comments made in this book. In desperation, as a drowning man, when forced to acknowledge my findings these selfsame persons will challenge my logic, my proofs, my conclusions.

As there is no place where it hurts more to be hit than in the pocketbook, I fully expect my professional qualifications, my purposes and even my basic integrity to be viciously slighted.

To all of this may I answer in advance: who I am, what I stand for, or anything else connected with me is of little importance with regards to the overall picture. What is important is the health, welfare, and lives of millions of persons. I readily admit that if you will work hard enough at it you may possibly be able to find minor flaws in certain arguments, processes of logic, procedures and so on. But nothing, I repeat nothing, can negate the incontrovertible fact that the basic cause of atherosclerosis and resulting clinical entities such as heart attacks and the most common forms of stroke is chlorine—the **chlorine** contained in "treated" municipal drinking water!

The fallacious cholesterol theory of atherosclerosis has been accepted for many years on the basis of most tenuous evidence. In retrospect we see that many most significant facts, especially those showing that atherosclerosis is almost exclusively a disease of modern Western Civilization, have been consciously or unconsciously ignored because they would cast serious doubt on the validity of the only widely if not universally-accepted (but only semi-plausible) theory presented until the advent of the present treatise.

On the other hand, we see that my Chlorine Theory accounts for not only all the widely accepted facts concerning atherosclerosis, but all the other facts and circumstances alluded to previously. Even if I could not produce experimental proofs to substantiate my claims, one would have to give very serious attention to my ideas on the basis of logical explanation of known facts alone. [My explanation of the previously unexplained situations regarding apparently anomalous occurrence of atherosclerotic diseases could be called the "circumstantial evidence" proof of my Chlorine Theory. Now, I know that at this point there will be many who will say "What we are dealing with is exact (medical) science, not art; we want reproducible, scientific experimental evidence." But medicine in general, by its very nature, cannot be completely reduced to pure science described in mathematical terms. It really is "the science and art of medicine", to use the old phrase, despite what some medical "researchers" who have never treated a live patient in their whole professional lives may insist. May I point out that with medical "science" it is often only the appearance of "black and white" so-called "scientific proofs" that we are shown. In fact, years ago when I was in medical school it was pointed out to us that ten years after we were to graduate that 50% of what we students had been taught as God-given medical facts and truths would be outdated or shown to be actually wrong! (And, of course, they were correct.) An example of the "grayness" of medical "research" is the fact that what is usually considered the ultimate of medical experimentation, that on actual, live animals, no matter how often repeated or what species used, give only general suggestions of what might possibly apply to human beings. (And this point is particularly true specifically with regards to animal experiments concerning cholesterol and the clogging of arteries called atherosclerosis.) Animals aren't human beings, and one must be especially careful in extrapolating results obtained from animal experimentation to humans. And on the other hand, under many circumstances human experiments may be impossible to perform because of moral restraints. Is someone going to propose that before they will accept my Chlorine Theory of atherogenesis that chlorine be given in extremely high doses (e.g. Vietnam War combat area levels of 20 to 30 times usual civilian municipal water residual concentrations?) to human volunteers for at least several years, with coronary angiography and/or luminal ultrasound being done before and after? Are these same cholesterol theory proponents themselves going to volunteer for such an experiment? Why not? After all, if residual chlorine in drinking water is, as they claim, absolutely harmless, absolutely unrelated to the development of atherosclerosis, how could they care if they drink water with 50 or 100 ppm (parts per million) of residual chlorine? Oh, such highly chlorinated water would be a bit raunchy tasting, but the Korean War and Vietnam War combat soldiers drank water with at least that level of chlorine every day. (In the field during combat operations in the U.S. Army, the "low man on totem pole" was in charge of putting in the hypochlorite in the water tank, and if anybody got sick from germs in the water he would have been in big trouble. So the universal pattern {without any testing} was, "If a little is good, more is better." The drinking water provided by the U.S. Army was yellow with chlorine, and the chlorine fumes coming off were shockingly strong! I know, I was there.

You "medical researchers" claim that chlorinated water is 100% safe, that chlorine does not cause atherosclerosis or anything else. I'm not asking you to do anything but drink anything or do anything else than what our soldiers had to do. You insist that chlorinated water can't hurt anyone. So I'm simply asking you to merely make the "sacrifice" of nothing more than regularly drinking something you insist is perfectly harmless, not so good tasting but just like our soldiers did, to prove me wrong. Put your actions where your mouths are, literally. What I cannot hardly believe is that "medical researchers" and the medical profession and other proponents of the cholesterol theory have allowed me to shoot off my mouth about how wrong and stupid they are and how right I am regarding chlorine and atherosclerosis for over thirty years. Why don't they prove me wrong? Of course, this is a rhetorical question, because they can't prove me wrong! To reiterate the essence of what I have just said, **Korean and Vietnam combat war veterans were unintentional victims of this "ultimate" chlorine/atherosclerosis human experimentation, with results** of autopsies of such men killed in battle versus well-known results of similar autopsies of civilian men the same age (e.g. killed in auto accidents) **being absolute proof of my claims! The ultimate, final "proof" of my "Chlorine Theory"** of atherogenesis, of chlorine in drinking water being the specific cause of heart attacks and most strokes, **was actually performed decades ago!**]

But disregarding the fact that with the ultimate (human) experiments in Korea and Vietnam proving my "Chlorine Theory" claims, I did do classical animal experimentation to try to satisfy those who would not believe me otherwise. And my results have been some of the most notable and specific ever presented in an entirely original publication on a medical subject.

[These experiments have been repeated, further experiments have been done over the years since the publication of the first edition of this book, all confirming my claims. The vested interests who oppose this book and its lifesaving message are always ready to parrot the old statement "more research is needed." And they tend to find an approving or at least acquiescent audience for this claim in as much as the general public has been brainwashed to believe that if the results of medical research does not emulate from the bowels of a famous "research institution" it cannot be valid (and probably is plain, old, "quackery".) They do not realize that these very "institutions" themselves have vested interests in the *status quo*, and, at least in the case of chlorine causing atherosclerosis are actually a very significant part of the problem instead of providing the answers to such!

For those scientifically vacuous individuals, whether lay or professional, who pick up the "more research is needed" mantra, may I point out that if chlorination of water supplies was under the auspices of the U.S. Food and Drug Administration they could have been required to ban chlorination of water supplies on an emergency basis years ago—no later than 1983 when the first U.S. Environmental Protection Agency reports confirming my claims became available. (See EPA letter dated March 24, 1986, signed by Donald J. Ehreth, as proof of the EPA's knowledge of the dangers of chlorine at the administrative level; experimental studies preceded such by several years.) It could have been banned like any drug discovered to have a previously unrecognized potentially serious or life-threatening side effect. The Food and Drug Administration places the responsibility for definite proof of safety on the sellers of the drugs, and is not required to wait for results of "more research" to act under such circumstances. They order the drug to be recalled immediately, and then the company that has been selling it (or anybody else) can do "more research" until the cows come home. But in the meantime they are not allowed to experiment on the unsuspecting public!

The cholesterol theory proponents have had not 30 days, not thirty weeks, but thirty years to prove me wrong. They have failed miserably and completely to do so. I must insist that my Chlorine Theory of atherosclerosis is much too important ("Coronary disease and atherosclerosis account for half of the reasons that people die today." —William P. Castelli, M.D., Medical Director of the Framingham {Mass.} Heart Study, "Cholesterol as a Cardiac Risk Factor", Doctors

Mart, Vol. 12, #4, 1988.) to let languish in obscurity by the repeated delaying tactics of mewling "more research is needed." What more could possibly be needed that what I reveal in this book, confirmed by the U.S. EPA's own studies?

Contrary to what might be suggested by my above comments, I am not demanding that chlorine in water supplies be banned immediately as a dangerous drug (which, of course, it is—the most dangerous of all drugs in terms of total number of persons injured or killed), but that the public be warned that present technology does not exist to immediately provide poison-free drinking water at the tap in the U.S. for everyone and that therefore it is the responsibility of each and every individual family to immediately protect themselves from the slow but inexorable ravages of chlorine ingestion with at least chlorine-free bottled, "spring" or distilled water, or basic filtration/treatment in the home and workplace to remove chlorine from tap water. (Unlike when the first edition of this book was produced, the logistics of providing chlorine-free water should not be a problem at all today. In some areas {e.g. California} a majority of persons are already drinking filtered or bottled water, as well as other chlorine-free drinks such as soda pop, fruit drinks and many other beverages. This fact is undoubtedly the otherwise not understood reason why there has been a drop in the incidence of heart attacks in America over the past couple decades.)

If at this point you are unconvinced enough to question the basic validity of my conclusions, let me make the following statement: I hereby make an unqualified challenge to all concerned to repeat my proofs—and expand on them. (The basic chicken experiment proof can be duplicated for a few hundred dollars. You wouldn't even need a research grant.) After you have done this you may criticize me as you see fit. Obviously, you will have "seen the light' and have realized that I have been correct all the time.

In closing, I want to parry one other possible criticism of me and my claims. There will be some who will insist that presenting this fantastic concept of the deadliness of chlorine in producing heart attacks and strokes to the general public without large-scale scientific "proof" performed in many independent laboratories is "premature." [The more recent "politically-correct" phrase would be to say "more research is needed."] To this just let me ask if it is proper to delay and let people die when they can live? My responsibilities as a physician are to my patients and society at large, not to certain special interest groups concerned about their own prestige and pocketbooks.

[I should note at this point that the U.S. government, specifically the people at the Health Effects Research Laboratory of the United States Environmental Protection Agency at Cincinnati, Ohio, have specifically confirmed my Chlorine Theory of Atherogenesis, by means of primate and other animal experiments, and have even performed definitive studies to "understand this phenomenon on the molecular and cellular level." (See letter reproduced in this book, signed by J. Peter Bercz, Ph.D.) This means that the U.S. government had produced their own definitive proof of my claims before 1987. My "Chlorine Theory" has not been a "theory" at all for more than a decade and a half, it is *incontrovertible fact!*]

Chapter 14

Future Avenues Of Research—Unanswered Questions

Many think that given enough money for medical research any disease can be licked, the time needed being inversely related to the quantity of funds made available. As their most notable example, they proudly point to the conquering of poliomyelitis ("polio') to support this assumption. (The large "foundations" have purposefully fostered this misconception, for obvious selfish reasons.)

Unfortunately, this line of thinking is totally fallacious. With polio the breakthrough in thinking (ie. the theory behind immunization as exemplified by smallpox vaccinations) had been accomplished more than 150 years before the finally successful practical program developing the Salk and then the Sabin oral vaccines. Conquering of the scourge of polio, because no new and original thinking was involved, was indeed a simple matter of money. Enough funding allowed multiple trial-and-error experiments to finally discover 1. an acceptable medium wherein to successfully grow the viruses, and 2. proper method of attenuation of the virus thus produced to create a usable and effective vaccine.

In contrast, any medical research situation wherein the breakthrough in thinking has not been accomplished is doomed to failure or at least most mediocre and ineffective results. How can anyone find a cure for cancer when no two researchers can really agree as to what cancer even is? ["Cancer" probably represents a large group of superficially similar disease processes with very significant differences. Just as no one antibiotic works for all infectious diseases, so it appears that no single treatment or even type of treatment can ever work for all "cancer." Unlike with polio (or my discovery of the specific cause of atherosclerotic diseases, mainly heart attack and stroke), no great individual genius is going to get the credit and maybe the Nobel Prize for single-handedly "licking cancer."] Yet brazen stories of imminent success regarding a potential "cure" for

71

cancer are periodically fed to the news media to keep the flow of donations and Federal grants coming.

Although this book explains in some detail the etiology (causation) of atherosclerosis [and its complications of heart attack and stroke] as being the direct result of chlorine ingestion, the exact mechanism of development of the plaques remains obscure. We now realize that atherosclerosis cannot occur [in otherwise healthy people] to a clinically significant degree in the absence of chlorine ingestion, but as yet have no idea as to the exact way chlorine acts in the body to produce the disease manifestations. Is it a straightforward process wherein the chlorine causes a simple deposition of normally-occurring cholesterol in the intima [inner lining] of arteries? Or a vastly complex mechanism involving multiple interactions of the body's whole biochemical system? [On December 17, 1986, Dr. J. Peter Bercz (United States Environmental Protection Agency toxicologist) phoned me at my Carsonville, Michigan medical office and (as alluded to in his follow-up letter of January 15, 1987—see copy printed in front pages of this book) went into great detail as to the exact biochemical mechanism of atherosclerosis they had worked out—from chlorine reacting with saliva to produce special chemical compounds through to the end deposition of material in the lining of arteries resulting in the actual physical plaques of atherosclerosis. The "We are now beginning to disassemble—" sentence in this letter to me refers to this biochemical mechanism.

[Today, the mechanism of development of the atheromas that cause clogging of the arteries is thought (by orthodox medical researchers) to be initiated by "cholesterol oxide" penetrating and being deposited inside the endothelium of such arteries. This foreign material (cholesterol oxide) does not normally exist in nature and therefore represents a form of "foreign body", which is consequently phagocytized (eaten up) by monocytes (white blood cells.) Instead of taking care of the situation, this process of phagocytosis results in the development of "foam cells", the initial evidence of atherosclerosis. Later these areas of "foam cells" are "organized" by muscle and other cells into mature atheromas that block the insides of the arteries. I just pointed out that cholesterol oxide is not a chemical normally found in bodies; it is the result of normal cholesterol (and doesn't matter if it is endogenous {made by the body itself} or exogenous {from ingested foodstuffs}) being oxidized by free chlorine from drinking water, chlorine being one of the most powerful oxidizing agents known to man! Therefore, as I have said for decades, the specific cause of atherosclerosis and resulting heart attacks and strokes is not cholesterol itself, a normal and very important chemical compound of the body, but the man-made, extremely harsh and powerful chemical oxidizing agent, chlorine from ingesting "treated" drinking water!]

These questions are of great interest because they could provide a clue as to whether existing disease is reversible and/or possibly even a method could be developed to promote such reversal.

Another question in my mind is the existence and significance of obstruction of the microcirculation proposed in this book. The chicken experiments certainly suggest most strongly the possibility of this kind of component of the action of chlorine in the body.

Conservative medical science acknowledges the existence of a disease entity called arteriosclerotic heart disease (abbreviated ASHD) which results in a weak, enlarged heart predisposed to arrhythmias and failure. This term seems to refer to a disease process quite separate from classical coronary heart disease involving closing of the lumen of the specific coronary or heart arteries. Is this ASHD a result of impairment of the micro-circulation caused by chlorine, an effect quite distinct from the chlorine-induced atheromatous plaque formation in the coronary arteries?

Are some cases of senile dementia really a combination disease with a single etiology, ie. chlorine? Is the blood flow to the brain impaired not only by the develop-ment of partially-obstructing atherosclerotic plaques in the arteries feeding the brain, by repeated embolism of small parts of arterial plaque resulting in "mini-strokes" ("multi-infarct dementia"), but also by a direct impairment of the microcirculation of the brain itself—another and distinct result of chlorine ingestion? I would think that the effects of ingested chlorine on the microcirculation of the brain would be a more likely cause of, or at least contributing factor to, Alzheimer's disease than something like the proposed ingested aluminum etiology of such.

Other unanswered questions include the mystery of why and how pre-menopausal women are protected from the deleterious effects of chlorine in causing atherosclerosis and resultant diseases. [I find it amazing how our communication media and therefore the general populace seems totally ignorant of the simple fact that menstruating women (without complicating diseases such as diabetes mellitus, hypertension, or systemic lupus erythematosis) are essentially 100% protected from any clogging of the arteries by atherosclerosis and therefore all heart attacks and strokes based on such process. In my clinical practice I see young, healthy women (who have been taken in by the continuing massive propaganda campaign of the cholesterol theory proponents) avoiding perfectly healthy foods such as red meat and eggs in the false belief that they are somehow protecting themselves from possible future atherosclerosis and heart attacks/ strokes! Such foolishness!

Chapter 15

Your Duty As An Interested Citizen

"The reception accorded to Jenner's work (the introduction of vaccination against smallpox) was the same as that usually accorded to great humane innovations. A few people received it with great acclaim, a somewhat greater number opposed it violently, and the vast majority were indifferent."

"Devils, Drugs and Doctors"
by Howard W. Haggard, M.D.

[In the first edition of this book I was ingenuous enough to ask my readers to write their Congressmen and Senators to demand that this Chlorine Theory be given proper consideration, that experiments be done to confirm (or refute) my claims. No, I do not apologize for such naivete. After all, Mr. Ralph Nader is on record as stating (*The Nader Report*, 1988), "The only remaining hurdle to attaining pure, safe drinking water in the United States is political. When sufficiently large numbers of people have been alerted to the health threat of toxics in their drinking water and demand action, the problem will be solved." Unfortunately, the hard, cold world of experience has made me somewhat of a cynic regarding the possibility of a sufficient number of persons demanding action, and legislators' usual responses to such demands which are inevitably meaningless form letters.

Yes, write your Congressmen and Senators, demand action. But in the meantime do as I have personally done for decades, protect your health and future by refusing to drink a single drop of chlorinated tapwater! (After avoiding all chlorinated water—drinking, shower or bath, and otherwise—for a while, you will be surprised at how sensitive you will become in detecting chlorinated water.

The average glass of water placed in front of you at a restaurant will almost make you retch!)]